SPIRITUAL PARTNERSHIP

Guide to Gary Zukav's Books

Each book is a stand-alone experience. They are all perfect starting points, so use your intuition.

The Dancing Wu Li Masters
An Overview of the New Physics
(1979)

Soul to Soul
Communications from the Heart (2007)

Thoughts from The Seat of the Soul
Meditations for Souls in Process (1994)

Soul Stories
(2000)
Illustrates some ideas in
The Seat of the Soul,
and more, with stories

The Seat of the Soul
(1989)
The key book—about soul, evolution, and authentic power

The Heart of the Soul
Emotional Awareness (2001)
(with Linda Francis)
In-depth explanation, experiential
learning, and practical applications

The Mind of the Soul
Responsible Choice (2003)
(with Linda Francis)
In-depth explanation, experiential
learning, and practical applications

Thoughts from The Heart of the Soul
**Meditations for
Emotional Awareness** (2002)

Self-Empowerment Journal
**Companion to
The Mind of the Soul** (2003)

Spiritual Partnership
The Journey to Authentic Power
(2010)
An in-depth guide to creating authentic
power and spiritual partnerships

SPIRITUAL PARTNERSHIP

The Journey to Authentic Power

GARY ZUKAV

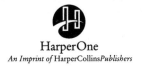

HarperOne
An Imprint of HarperCollinsPublishers

Harper One

SPIRITUAL PARTNERSHIP: *The Journey to Authentic Power.* Copyright © 2010 by Gary Zukav. All rights reserved. Printed in the United States of America. No part of this book may be used or reproduced in any manner whatsoever without written permission except in the case of brief quotations embodied in critical articles and reviews. For information address HarperCollins Publishers, 10 East 53rd Street, New York, NY 10022.

HarperCollins books may be purchased for educational, business, or sales promotional use. For information please write: Special Markets Department, HarperCollins Publishers, 10 East 53rd Street, New York, NY 10022.

HarperCollins Web site: http://www.harpercollins.com

HarperCollins®, 👑®, and HarperOne™ are trademarks of HarperCollins Publishers

FIRST EDITION

Library of Congress Cataloging-in-Publication Data

Zukav, Gary.
    Spiritual partnership : the journey to authentic power / by Gary Zukav. — 1st ed.
        p. cm.
    ISBN 978-0-06-145850-7
    1. Spiritual life—New Age Movement. 2. Spirituality. 3. Interpersonal relations—Religious aspects. I. Title.
    BP605.N48Z8539   2010
    299'.93—dc22   2009046574

        10   11   12   13   14   RRD(H)   10   9   8   7   6   5   4   3   2   1

This book is dedicated to spiritual partners
and potential spiritual partners everywhere

Contents

WHAT

HOW

Prologue
Change, Possibilities, Power

This is a book about change, the biggest change possible or imaginable—change bigger than the discovery of fire, bigger than the invention of the wheel, bigger than the origin of cultures, the birth of religions, the rise of nation-states, and the impacts of science. It is bigger than anything that has come before and so big that it is not possible to envision what could come after or when.

This is a book about possibilities. Experiences, insights, motivations, and creations beyond our ability to imagine only a few years ago now call to us, beckoning us to new destinations and yet more new possibilities. All is new and fresh, like a blank page awaiting words, a canvas inviting the first brushstroke. In the past others have glimpsed, and sometimes explored, these new possibilities, but now everyone is beginning to see or sense them. We have crossed a threshold and there is no turning back. There is no way to turn back.

This is a book about power. The old kind of power—the ability to manipulate and control—now produces only violence and destruction. This is a real surprise, because the old power enabled us and our ancestors to survive. Like good medicine suddenly turned bad, it is now poison. We used to take it to stay alive. Now we need to avoid it to stay healthy. A new kind of power—authentic power—has become the new good medicine, and we need it to become healthy, nurturing, and whole.

Change, possibilities, and power that we could not have imagined are reshaping the entire human experience. New values, goals, and intentions are everywhere appearing like grass in the spring. This grass is growing quickly, and wherever it grows, beauty appears. With it come fields of flowers and vast forests. A new and surprising world is emerging in new and surprising ways. We are all students in a new school, explorers in new territory, and pioneers in a new human experience.

This unprecedented transformation in human experience has two parts. We can call them Process A and Process B. Process A is happening automatically, so to speak. No one needs to do anything to make Process A happen. Process A is occurring in millions of individuals, and soon Process A will occur in all humans. Process B is a different story. It requires choice. Specifically, *you* must choose to make Process B happen or it will not happen in you. Even if others choose to make Process B happen in themselves, Process B will not happen in you until you choose to make it happen. In short, (1) Process A is happening to everyone, or soon will, and there is nothing that you or anyone else can do about it; (2) Process B is happening only to individuals who choose to make it happen in themselves; no one else can make it happen in them; and they cannot make it happen in anyone else.

Let's give Process A and Process B names. Process A is the expansion of human perception beyond what we can see, hear, taste, touch, and smell. It is a very big deal. Process A is seeing for yourself that the world is larger than you thought—much larger—and also different than you could have imagined. Before Process A occurs, your perceptions of the world are confined to what your five senses tell you about it. After Process A occurs, your five senses continue to tell you about the world and, in addition, you experience more. The "more" is sometimes difficult to describe to individuals who have not yet experienced Process A, but actually, millions of individuals have already experienced Process A or are experiencing it and haven't realized it yet.

Process A allows you to know things about others that your five senses cannot tell you, for example, that someone is going to call you just before she calls, that your daughter in another city has been in an accident, that your grandparent is passing on, that you should avoid driving until you check the brakes on your car, and so on. In other words, Process A involves intuition in a big way. Process A also allows you to experience yourself in new ways, for example, as more than your mind and your body. It reveals your life as purposeful and calls you to your purpose like water calls a thirsty man. Process A allows you to encounter meaning in unexpected ways, for example, a brief experience that everything is perfect, or a feeling of connection with a stranger. Process A allows you to see from an impersonal perspective. From that perspective, all of your experiences—even the most painful—serve your spiritual development and the spiritual development of those around you. They provide exactly what you need to develop the strength, compassion, and wisdom to give the gifts that you were born to give.

Process A is an expanded awareness that includes not only the perceptual system of the five senses but also a second system that detects intelligence, compassion, and wisdom that are real but not physical. This system allows you to experience nonphysical reality in many ways, including those just mentioned. Process A is multisensory perception. This is the great transformation in human consciousness that is currently emerging throughout the human species. Within a few generations, all humans will be multisensory. They will experience not only the domain of space, time, matter, and duality that has been the totality of experience for most humans since the origin of humanity, but also nonphysical domains and dynamics that affect us and that we affect.

This brings us to Process B. Process B is bringing the new potential that comes with Process A into your life. Multisensory perception (Process A) changes your perception, but it does not change you. It shows you things that you could not see before, but it does not make you use your new knowledge. It illuminates dynamics that you could not see—dynamics that you can apply to change your life and world permanently for the better—but it does not require you to apply them. It reveals your creative power, but it does not make you create wisely. On the contrary, you will continue to create as you have in the past until you choose otherwise. If you are angry, for example, Process A (multisensory perception) will not make you less angry. It also will not create different consequences for you than acting with anger has created in the past. People will still avoid you, still be intimidated by you, still refuse to be vulnerable with you, and you will still be isolated, lonely, longing for meaningful relationships, and angry.

Process B is experiencing and changing in yourself the interior sources of your painful emotions (such as anger, jealousy, vengefulness, and so on), obsessive thoughts (such as judging others or yourself, longing for someone or something to change your life, and so on), compulsive activities (such as workaholism, perfectionism, and so on), and addictive behaviors (such as overeating, smoking, drinking alcohol, using drugs, watching pornography, gambling, and so on). It is also experiencing and cultivating in yourself the interior sources of your pleasing emotions (such as gratitude, contentment, appreciation, and awe of Life). In short, Process B is creating the fulfilling and joyful life that is calling to you.

This takes work, but choosing Process B can produce almost instantaneous results in your life. In other words, choosing Process B can fundamentally change your life in a very short time. This does not mean that you become a radically different person the first or second time you engage in Process B. Process B is not that simple or easy. However, each change that you make in yourself as you engage in Process B is fundamentally transformative. The first change is fundamentally transformative, no matter how small it may appear. The second change is fundamentally transformative, and so forth. Process B is incremental. It happens choice by choice, and each choice that you make moves you in a new direction toward a new and healthy goal—a personality whose experiences are so dramatically different that you cannot always foresee what they will be.

Process B requires you to choose words and deeds, moment by moment, that will create joyful and constructive consequences *even when painful or violent emotions roar through you.* Process B is changing your life with the force of your own will, guided by your own awareness, with intentions that you consciously choose, assisted by the compassion and wisdom of the Universe experienced in personal and meaningful ways. This transformation is more than change toward a better or more healthy life. It is transformation toward the highest, most noble, healthy, and grounded part of you. That is your soul.

In other words, Process B is finding and changing all the parts of your personality that do not intend what your soul intends, and finding and cultivating all the parts of your personality that do intend what your soul intends. Your soul intends harmony, cooperation, sharing, and reverence for Life. Each time you create with one of these intentions, you create authentic power—a life of meaning, fulfillment, gratitude, vitality, creativity, and joy. Process B is creating authentic power.

Without Process A (multisensory perception) happening to everyone, Process B (creating authentic power) would not be possible for anyone. Process B is aligning your personality with your soul, but your five senses cannot detect your soul. The soul is an interesting idea to some five-sensory individuals, but it is not experientially meaningful to any of them. Now millions of individuals are experiencing multisensory perception (Process A), and they are changing their lives because of it (Process B). You are experiencing multisensory perception or you would not find this book interesting or valuable. The ideas in it have no appeal to intellects that are informed by the five senses alone, but they call to all hearts that are informed by multisensory perception.

Multisensory perception and authentic power are the two defining characteristics of the transformation in human consciousness that is now under way. The first emerges without effort, affects all perception, and reveals new dimensions of experience. The second awaits your commitment, courage, compassion, and conscious communications and actions to bring it into your life. The first is a wondrous gift from the Universe. You must create the second.

Multisensory perception does not impair your choice. Multisensory individuals are as free to pursue external power (the old kind of power) as they are to create authentic power, but the choice to pursue external power now leads only to violence and destruction—emotional violence and destruction between individuals (at the least), and physical violence and destruction between religions, cultures, and nations. There are no redeeming benefits to the choice of external power. There are no benefits to it at all.

Five-sensory humans evolve by surviving. Multisensory humans evolve by growing spiritually. This dramatic difference requires dramatically different relationships. The new type of relationship for multisensory humans who are evolving through creating authentic power is spiritual partnership. A spiritual partnership is a partnership between equals for the purpose of spiritual growth. It attracts multisensory humans who are creating authentic power as much as old-type relationships attracted five-sensory humans who were pursuing external power. The purpose, nature, and function of spiritual partnerships are different. The dynamics of spiritual partnerships and the experiences that spiritual partners cocreate are different. This new type of relationship is as inseparable from emerging multisensory humans who are creating authentic power as old-type relationships were from five-sensory humans who pursued external power.

Creating authentic power requires relationships of substance and depth. You cannot grow spiritually until you have the courage to enter into meaningful and significant relationships. In other words, spiritual partnerships are a necessary part of Process B. Every encounter provides you an opportunity to create authentic power, but when your encounters include others who are also using their experiences to create authentic power, the potential for a spiritual partnership comes into being. Potential spiritual partners recognize the commitment, courage, compassion, and conscious communications and actions of one another. They naturally strive to support one another in creating authentic power and to receive the support of one another in creating authentic power. They journey toward the same goal, recognize fellow travelers, and learn from one another. Evolution now requires you to create a fulfilling and joyful life—to give the gifts that you were born to give—and spiritual partnerships bring you into cocreative interactions with others who are doing the same.

All of the books that I have written, or coauthored with my spiritual partner Linda Francis, are about authentic power. The first was *The Dancing Wu Li Masters: An Overview of the New Physics,* although I did not know it at the time. This book is about quantum physics, relativity, and quantum logic for people with no interest in science, but writing it introduced me for the first time to some experiences of authentic power. I did not know how to identify or articulate them, but I recognized these experiences as remarkable and wonderful, and I opened myself wide to them. The book won many awards and much praise as a popularization of science, but I believe that many of the people who read it (and still read it) are drawn to the connections between physical reality and consciousness that are unavoidable in some of the interpretations of the quantum theory, including the one that is used by most physicists. *The Dancing Wu Li Masters* was my first attempt at writing and my first inquiry into science, but more than that, it was my first gift to Life, and I am still receiving gifts in return.

The second book was about authentic power but without any vehicle, such as science. It shares all that I discovered about authentic power while and since writing *The Dancing Wu Li Masters*. It began as a three-volume product of the intellect called *Physics and Consciousness,* but ten years later it had become another gift of the heart, *The Seat of the Soul.* Some readers expected me to write a sequel to *The Dancing Wu Li Masters* about another pioneering field of science, such as genetics. I had reservations about disappointing them, but I could not remain in integrity without sharing this wonderful book. Like *The Dancing Wu Li Masters,* it changed my life, but in ways that I could not have imagined.

At the time I thought that I understood authentic power, but I had not yet realized that my understanding was not as deep as it would become and that understanding authentic power and creating an authentically powerful life are not identical. Eventually, Linda, whom I met after *The Seat of the Soul* was published, and I coauthored books on two of the tools for creating authentic power (*The Heart of the Soul: Emotional Awareness* and *The Mind of the Soul: Responsible Choice*). I also wrote two light-reading books with vignettes and examples of multisensory perception and authentic power (*Soul Stories* and *Soul to Soul: Communications from the Heart*), but in my heart I continued to long for another book to explain the creation of authentic power in clearer and clearer ways, to illustrate it, and to give readers concrete as well as conceptual examples of multisensory perception and how to create authentic power.

This is that book. *The Seat of the Soul* and *Spiritual Partnership* are both about Process A and Process B. *The Seat of the Soul* is about evolution, cause and effect, intuition, intention, responsibility, and trust, among other things, but it emphasizes Process A. It focuses on the electric experiences of becoming multisensory, cocreating with always-present nonphysical Teachers and guides, and partnering consciously with the compassionate and wise Universe. *Spiritual Partnership* is also about multisensory perception and authentic power, but it emphasizes Process B. It shows the Why, What, How, and Who of spiritual partnership and, therefore, of creating authentic power. Spiritual partnerships and creating authentic power are as inseparable as wisdom and patience. Without creating authentic power you cannot have spiritual partners, and without spiritual partners you cannot grow spiritually.

Creating authentic power is a process, not an event. It is the purpose of your life and the opportunity of your interactions. Authentic power is a journey, not a destination. It is a journey that few have taken before and that all of us are now required to complete as humanity transits from a five-sensory species that evolved by surviving into a multisensory species that evolves by growing spiritually. This book is a road map to creating authentic power. Refer to it at any point along the way. Read it to prepare for what lies ahead, and review it to understand what lies behind. Practice it to live joyfully wherever you are at this moment on the journey.

I am grateful to be on the journey with you.

Introduction

Relationships

A new type of relationship is emerging in the human experience. It is replacing all other forms of relationship, and this is good news. Previous types of relationships were designed for a human species that is dying. A new human species is being born, and we are part of it. It has its own requirements for relationships, its own values, and its own goals. Its potential is greater than the potential of the species that is disappearing, and its ability to contribute constructively to the human experience is far greater.

Millions of individuals are part of this new species, and millions more are becoming part of it. It expands daily because babies with new capabilities are born daily and also because millions of individuals are becoming aware of these same capabilities within themselves. You are one of those individuals or you would not be drawn to this book. *Spiritual* would be a concept to you, or a religion, or a belief system. You would think of *spirituality* in religious, poetic, or philosophical terms, or imagine it in terms of heavens, ascending to higher levels of experience (or being condemned to lower levels of experience). You would put a cross, a statue of the Buddha, an image of Krishna, a crystal, or a painting of radiant inspiration on your altar or mantel. You would recite mantras or prayers, chant or sing hymns, and take comfort in the companionship of colleagues who have discovered the same truth as you.

The new type of human relationship separates *spiritual* and *religious*. Spirituality is not a matter of conforming to tradition, complying with commandments, implementing instructions, or accepting the authority of others. It also does not have to do with buildings, ways of dressing, scriptures, and holy writings, although it does have to do with appreciating the holy in everything and striving to live accordingly. Last, spirituality does not have to do with judgment of others or yourself, but with discovering within yourself and transforming within yourself the interior causes of your painful experiences and destructive behaviors, and discovering within yourself and cultivating within yourself the interior causes of your joyful experiences and constructive behaviors.

The new type of relationship, the new understanding of spirituality, and the new human species are being born together and are designed for one another. The distinction between spirituality and religion is not apparent to the old human being, but it is becoming obvious to millions of individuals. Nevertheless, some confusion remains not only because the transformation from the old humanity to the new humanity is in progress and not yet complete, but also because many people who are religious are also spiritual, and the other way around, many people who are spiritual are also religious. This is a time of great transition when the old is falling away, the new is emerging, and for several generations the two will overlap as the influences of the old humanity and its values and goals wane and the influences of the new humanity with its different values and goals increase.

This process is irreversible, so attachments to the old humanity and its goals have no usefulness and, on the contrary, can create only painful experiences and consequences. How anguishing would it be to grieve the rising of the sun each morning, or the tide coming in or going out? What could that accomplish other than personal misery? The biggest occurrence in human history outside of the origin of humanity is under way, and we are part of it whether we accept it or reject it, welcome it or push it away, embrace it or resist it. A new human relationship dynamic is integral to that occurrence, and therefore, we can also accept or reject it, welcome or spurn it, but we cannot ignore it without consequences. Relationships are the most difficult human endeavors, and now that the nature of human relationships is changing, they are becoming even more difficult for those who ignore the change.

There are as many different relationships of the old type as there are shared goals. Business relationships are different from romantic relationships, which are different from relationships between classmates, relationships between neighbors, and relationships between parents and children. The relationship between you and your mechanic is different from the relationship between your physician and his office manager, although that relationship is more like your relationship with your accountant or mechanic. Property owners have relationships with renters; employees have relationships with coworkers and employers; and teachers have relationships with students.

The individuals within these relationships work to accomplish a shared goal. The relationships allow the individuals involved to accomplish goals that they could not accomplish by themselves. For example, election campaigns, corporations, and barn raisings are all products of this type of relationship. Some relationships are so impersonal that the connection between individuals within them is irrelevant, such as the relationship between a policeman directing traffic and the drivers he directs. Yet the participants together create what none can accomplish alone—a smooth flow of traffic. Some are mostly impersonal yet allow for mutual appreciation, such as a relationship between you and a clerk. In others, the connection between individuals becomes much more important, such as your relationships with your in-laws, although those relationships may or may not be intimate or substantive.

The goal of raising a healthy family or living together in mutually supportive ways requires much more focus on the connection between the individuals involved, because if that connection is missing or superficial, the goal cannot be attained. Board members can despise one another, which happens frequently; employees can compete with one another, which is common; and political allies can exploit one another, which they usually do, and still accomplish their shared goals. These relationships are difficult and painful, but they are functional. In fact, most relationships fall into this category. Countless marriages and domestic partnerships are painfully difficult, yet the individuals involved remain in them because they provide a sense of safety or at least familiarity that each partner fears losing, and in this way the partners accomplish a shared goal. Relationships in which partners focus on creating positive connections between themselves as well as on accomplishing their shared goal are the most challenging.

The function of all old-type relationships, from those in which connection between the participants is negligible to those in which it is central, is to manipulate or control circumstances (including other people) to attain a goal that the participants share—in other words, to change the external world, for example, to elect a mayor, organize a movement, or build a business. This type of relationship enables partners to buy a house together, have children, raise a family, keep each other from loneliness, or satisfy their emotional, psychological, physical, or sexual needs with each other. Their shared goal is always the reason for their relationship. When the goal is accomplished, or they fail to accomplish it, the relationship breaks apart. For example, an election campaign ends when an opponent wins and the campaigners separate; a business fails and the partners go their separate ways, or it succeeds and they sell the business and go their separate ways.

There are countless variations of this theme: A marriage partner realizes that her spouse cannot or is not willing to satisfy her psychological, physical, emotional, or sexual needs and divorces. An individual becomes a vegetarian, is "born again," begins to meditate, or adopts another religion and no longer seeks or accepts relationships with individuals who have not similarly changed. Any transition that makes an individual different in belief or appearance, or that creates a difference of values or goals, will end an old-type relationship, because the shared goal that underlies it is no longer there. Whether the shared goal is the security of sameness—such as skin color, belief, or language—or increased market share, a new board of supervisors, or a happy family, it is the reason for the relationship and the glue that holds it together. Without the shared goal, the relationship ceases to have meaning, mutual attraction among the participants diminishes, and the relationship disintegrates or is replaced with others that are more relevant.

Whatever the goal is, it determines who will be attractive as a potential partner and who will not, who will be welcome and who will be pushed away. Homogeneity is accepted, diversity is rejected. If the shared goal is acceptance, for example, individuals who do not speak, dress, act, or believe in the way that the relationship requires are not eligible for membership. An individual who wants a partner to support a future family will not consider someone who is unemployable or refuses to work. The director of a play will not consider individuals who cannot act, a business owner who needs a marketing director will not consider individuals who do not have that ability or aptitude, and so on.

The shared goal determines the participants in the relationship, and those participants are replaceable. One carpenter can be replaced with another, one campaign manager can be replaced with another, one volunteer can be replaced with another, and as many individuals have discovered, one spouse can be replaced with another.

Relationships of this type are familiar because we see them everywhere and experience them continually. They served the survival of the human species that is dying out, but they cannot support us now because the new species has perceptions and values that are very different from those of the old species. As more and more of us experience the new perceptions and values of the new human species, we begin to see ourselves and one another differently, our world differently, and the purpose of our lives differently. Our reason for being together changes, and therefore, the type of relationship that we create with one another changes. Old-type relationships are the means by which our species has survived and expanded to cover the Earth. However, they prevent spiritual growth.

This is significant, because we now evolve by growing spiritually. Spiritual growth is as necessary for us as sunshine is for a plant. We seek partners with whom we can grow spiritually rather than with whom we can accomplish common goals. Survival is not our only objective, or sufficient for us. We long for more, and as we strive for fulfillment we are redefining spirituality, relationship, and evolution.

The old humanity, evolution through survival, relationships designed to change circumstances, and religions are woven of the same fabric. They emerged together, and they are being replaced together by another fabric through which is woven the new humanity, evolution through spiritual growth, relationships designed for spiritual growth, and spirituality. The old fabric is unraveling. The new fabric is already out of the loom and becoming visible to more and more individuals.

Spirituality has to do with the soul and requires alignment with the most noble impulses of the human experience—harmony, cooperation, sharing, and reverence for Life. This goal cannot be brought into being for one person by another, or even by a collective of others. The spiritual development of an individual is not a barn raising made possible by helpful neighbors. Each individual is responsible for his or her own spiritual growth. Spirituality is a journey into self-awareness and self-responsibility. The old type of relationship helped the old humanity survive by focusing the attention of participants outward onto circumstances and people in order to change them. The new type of relationship enables us to grow spiritually by focusing our attention inward onto the interior causes of our painful experiences and destructive actions in order to change them, and onto the interior causes of our blissful experiences and constructive actions in order to cultivate them.

Old humans in search of spiritual growth escaped the distractions of circumstances and people by retreating into monasteries and nunneries, and from there into hermitages. The solitary meditator in a cell or cave became the icon of commitment to spiritual growth—expansion beyond the limitations of the five senses and the confines of culture and custom into the freedom of a life unbounded by fear. With the emergence of the new humanity, isolation has become counterproductive. It prevents the very interactions that are necessary for our spiritual development. Before, few individuals were interested in growing spiritually, and every relationship formed around a common goal. Now, millions of us are attracted to harmony, cooperation, sharing, and reverence for Life; within a few generations all humans will strive for spiritual growth; and we are already creating relationships that are quite different from the old type in order to support our spiritual development.

Relationships were necessary to the evolution of the old human species, and they are equally necessary to our evolution, but for significantly different reasons. Relationships helped the old species survive. They help us grow spiritually. As the values and perceptions of the new species emerge in millions of humans, relationships of the old type are becoming increasingly unsatisfactory. We are becoming increasingly interested in self-exploration, self-awareness, and self-mastery. Fulfillment, contentment, meaning, purpose, love, and the joy of contributing to

Life are taking precedence over issues such as career, lifestyle, and money.

We are finding it less and less satisfying to blame others for our painful experiences (no matter how much we still want to) than to discover within ourselves the causes of our painful experiences and change them. We are beginning to recognize the importance of our emotions and intentions, of what we do, what we say, and why. We are looking for connections between our choices and our experiences so that we can change our choices and, therefore, change our experiences. We are striving to be the kind of person we want others to be rather than to change others, and we are transforming our relationships at home, at work, and at play into relationships of the new type.

The terrain of human interaction is changing dramatically. Old-type relationships have no future, while relationships of the new type are appearing everywhere and in surprising ways. The scale of this change in the function, nature, and experience of relationship is enormous, but the reason behind it is even larger.

WHY

1

New Land, New Explorers

When the Vikings came to North America they were looking for plunder. Columbus was looking for a trade route. European colonialists sought land and riches. As they moved across this continent they took by force what they desired and impoverished the people they encountered. They accomplished what they intended, but none foresaw that their drive to dominate would destroy not only Native cultures but also the environment that supports us all.

The American settlers—originally oppressed people who won their freedom with blood and valor—became oppressors themselves, foraging as they forced themselves across North America, sometimes allying with colonialists and sometimes battling them. Their impact on the environment at first was small. They felled trees, cultivated fields, and built cities, but endless forests, clean water, and virgin prairies continually appeared before them.

That soon changed. The industrial revolution transformed the cultural and terrestrial landscape of the continent. Telegraph, railroads, automobiles, aircraft, computers, and spacecraft followed one another in close order, all appearing within two centuries. The population grew and then expanded exponentially as more settlers, slaves from Africa, and workers from Europe, Asia, and later, Latin America merged into a large, and then huge, consuming collective that threatened the ability of the continent to support its survival. That is where we are today, the inheritors of an expanding devastation that reflects the consciousness of the original settlers of North America.

This is the story of my land, the history of my parents and their ancestors who came to it and contributed to its transformation in ways that they could not have anticipated. They did not consider the consequences of their decisions, individual and collective, as they strove to achieve countless goals with the same consciousness that the original immigrants brought to this continent—the intention to control it and dominate it.

This is also the story of my Earth and the larger collective of cultures and individuals that, long before the Vikings came to North America, were creating the same consequences with the same consciousness. Nations, religions, industrialization, and militarization appeared on the pages of human history, transforming it into a chronicle of conflict and exploitation. Today the destructive impact on North America of its expanding population mirrors the larger destructive impact on the Earth of the expanding human population. In other words, this story is not one of place and time, but of *consciousness.*

A consciousness is the way that we experience ourselves and each other. It includes much more than emotions and thoughts. For example, we see some people as friends and others as enemies. The five senses cannot tell you whether a person is a friend or an enemy. They show you what your mother looks like to you, sounds like to you, and how her touch feels to you, but your experiences with your mother tell you that she is a friend, and your emotions reflect your experiences. When you see enemies, or think about them, you feel painful emotions, and when you see or think about friends, you feel pleasing emotions. When you encounter someone you do not know, what you think about that person creates your experiences. If you assume that she is a friend you will have different experiences than if you assume that she is an enemy. All of this is part of a consciousness, and yet there is even more.

A consciousness is like a bowl. The bowl is always full. Sometimes it has flowers in it, and at other times it has weapons.

Sometimes it has pictures of friends and people you love, and at other times it has experiences that terrify you. Everything that you see, everything that you imagine, thoughts about what you see and imagine, and your emotions are all in the bowl. Everything that you experience—such as your aspirations, fears, joy, disappointments, gratitude, and terror—appears in the bowl. There is no limit to what the bowl can contain. Its contents are always changing. The bowl does not change.

Imagine a bowl that is always filled with something from your kitchen. Sometimes it is filled with breakfast cereal, at other times with chicken soup, and at other times with spaghetti and sauce. Sometimes it is filled with fruit, then with salad, and then with onion peels. It is never empty. Although the things you can find in the bowl continually change, the bowl remains the same. If it was white and round when it was filled with cereal, it will be white and round when it is filled with salad. The bowl is different from the content of the bowl. Consciousness is like the bowl. The number of experiences that it can contain is unlimited, but no matter what is in it, the consciousness itself does not change.

Our collective experiences are also part of the content of consciousness. For example, a few centuries ago the world seemed flat and the sun appeared to revolve around the Earth. Everyone agreed with these ideas because they were obvious, but they are not obvious now. Students and scholars study differences between our experiences and the experiences of our ancestors, but our ancestors lived those differences. They actually experienced the world in ways other than we do. Paganism, the Greek gods, the religions of the past two and a half millennia, and writing each changed the content of the bowl. The development of mathematics, science, art, architecture, and governance also changed the content of the bowl, and changed it again and again as they evolved. The idea of progress, the rule of law, democracy, and technology are some of the latest changes in the content, yet through all these changes the bowl remained the same.

It is not possible to be born without a consciousness any more than it is possible to be born without a body. Every body is unique, yet each is recognizable as a body no matter how different it is from your own. Even if a body does not have all its limbs or eyes, or is shaped very differently or moves very differently than other bodies, it is recognizable as a body. What appears to be the same body over time is actually an entirely new body many times over the course of a lifetime. Old cells die and are replaced with new cells, which in turn die and are replaced. Infants grow into toddlers, children, adults, and elders. Limber bones and muscles become stronger, reaction times and endurance improve dramatically, and then deteriorate as the body approaches the end of its existence and changes dramatically again. Limbs or organs may be lost, damaged, or absent from birth, yet throughout its lifetime, young or old, whole or damaged, the body remains, and everyone knows and understands this. The body is the container, and the content of the container is always changing.

The bowl that is consciousness is like a body that can always be recognized anywhere and anytime because its basic form is like all others. Consciousness also has a basic form that is everywhere and always the same. No matter how much the content of the bowl changes, certain experiences never change. They are shared by every individual, regardless of where she comes from, what language she speaks, or what she believes. Everyone who has a consciousness has these experiences, and since everyone has a consciousness, everyone has these experiences. They are not limited to certain cultures or individuals. They cannot be ignored, dismissed, or denied. Unlike obvious experiences (such as the Earth is flat) that can be replaced by different obvious experiences (such as the Earth is round), these experiences are permanent. From birth to death and generation to generation they remain, underlying all other experiences. They are the common denominator of all peoples from all places in all times.

They are the essential human experiences that have not changed since the beginning of humanity.

These experiences are determined by the bowl, not by the content of the bowl. They show us the nature of the bowl, not the content of the bowl. This is territory that does not change. It is well known to every human because we all live in it. In fact, we have been exploring it since the very first human. This is the territory of the five senses. If a round bowl is filled with water, the water can never take the shape of a square. No matter what fills this bowl (consciousness), it can take only the shape of the bowl—what we can see, hear, taste, touch, and smell.

Whatever we imagine or think about, we can imagine or think about only in terms of the five senses. Sky, oceans, streets, mountains, and friends all appear in terms of the five senses. Hot, cold, large, small, quick, and slow appear in terms of the five senses. Generous, cruel, kind, frightened, and loving are meaningful only in terms of the five senses. Thoughts and emotions are understandable only in terms of the five senses (they appear as products of hormones and brain activities). Even abstract mathematics, which contains symbols that do not correspond to anything that we can imagine, has no value apart from what it can tell us about things that we can think about and describe in terms of the five senses.

Human experience throughout its history, with a few very notable exceptions, has been limited to the perceptions of the five senses. Even when we think about eternity and the infinite, we are forced to think in terms of the five senses because we cannot imagine anything eternal or infinite except as more of the same lasting forever or extending forever. We cannot even imagine forever except in terms of the five senses. When we think about heaven or hell, we imagine them, too, in terms of the five senses. In fact, we cannot think about *anything* except in terms of the five senses.

The five senses and the intellect work together. The five senses provide information, such as what color something is, how close or far away it is, how fast or slowly it is moving, how loud or quiet it is, and whether a person is smiling or scowling. The intellect uses this information. It compares, analyzes, deduces, and concludes. Coupled with the five senses, it allows us to accomplish what no other species has been able to accomplish—manipulation and control of our environment. For example, we know not only how to avoid danger, but also how to grow food, heat a house, build computers, use the internet, and much more. Everything that we have been able to accomplish since the first human has been because of the intellect. Many other forms of life, such as our fellow mammals, have five senses but they do not have intellects like we do. Only we can build boats and airplanes, spacecraft and telephones, tractors and highways, and apartment buildings.

All of these creations and our thoughts about them and every other experience that we can have are the content of consciousness—the things that fill the bowl. The bowl always comes in the shape of the five senses. Countless experiences come and go, continually changing the content of the container, but the container remains the same, day after day, year after year, millennium after millennium. Human history chronicles the exploration of everything that the five senses can detect, and the use of everything that the five senses detect to survive and become comfortable. Art, science, poetry, military conquests, religious conquests, agriculture, philosophy, ethics, and engineering all spring from the exploration of our world and our understanding of it. Our experiences of our world are the experiences of the five senses, and our understanding of those experiences is the product of the intellect.

Human experience appears dynamic and continually changing, but it has not really changed at all since the first human. The consciousness that created our experiences of the Earth—flat or round, stationary at the center of the universe or revolving around a minor star—and all else has itself remained constant from its origin until recently.

Now the shape of the bowl has changed, and nothing that we learned before the bowl changed shape can help us navigate the territory that we are encountering for the first time. A huge change is occurring not only in what we experience, but in what we *can* experience. Human consciousness is expanding beyond the limitations of the five senses. In some cases, it is exploding beyond them. The intellect cannot help us make sense of these new perceptions, or even articulate them, because it is designed to work with the five senses. Although we cannot describe or picture our new experiences, they are very real.

Not everyone is encountering these new experiences at the same time or at the same rate. Some catch glimpses of meaning in ordinary situations that they did not see before; for others, extraordinary experiences, such as unlikely coincidences, seem natural. Some people realize that their values are changing or have already changed. Others are frightened by what they experience, and they pretend that they have not experienced anything. All of this is happening very fast from an evolutionary perspective. Within a few generations, no one in the human species will be limited to the perceptions of the five senses. Our grandchildren's children will not be able to imagine anyone whose perception is confined to the five senses any more than we can imagine anyone without a consciousness.

The five senses are different aspects of a single sensory system. That system is designed to detect anything that is physical—anything that can be seen, heard, touched, smelled, or tasted. Now each of us in our own time and way is acquiring another sensory system. We are becoming multisensory. This second system detects wisdom and compassion, intelligence and design, purpose and existence that are not physical. Its perceptions do not replace the familiar perceptions of the five senses, but they give them a new dimension something like color gives a new dimension to black-and-white images, but they provide much more than that.

Some people are discovering that they know things about others, including strangers, that their five senses did not tell them, such as whether or not that person is kind or happy, experiencing a tragedy, getting married, or getting divorced. They have hunches, such as the idea to avoid a certain street at night, return to lock the door, or buy a certain book, and afterward regret not paying attention to them, or appreciate that they did. Familiar coincidences, such as a friend calling at the moment that we think of her, seem normal. Caring people still remain caring, and impatient people remain impatient; coworkers are still angry or compassionate; the seasons still come and go; infants are born and the elderly die, but our experiences of these things become richer and different. We sense that our lives are more meaningful than we ever thought. The content of the bowl is different than it could have been in the past because the shape of the bowl is different for the first time in the history of the bowl.

Our view of ourselves as physical and limited in duration is being replaced by experiences of ourselves as souls as well as bodies and minds, as immortal beings as well as mortal personalities. This is the biggest change. We are beginning to glimpse that neither consciousness nor responsibility ends at death, and that everything we experience holds out to us the potential of spiritual development. The events of our lives appear meaningful instead of random.

Our experiences of the Universe are changing. Instead of understanding it as inert (dead) and consciousness as unexplainable and temporary, we are beginning to experience the Universe, or at least think of it, as living, wise, and compassionate. A larger picture of Life is becoming visible in which we are not separate from each other or anything. We are not separate from the stars or the sand on the beach, from those we love or those we hate.

When I moved to a ranch in a rural valley in northern California, I brought with me habits that I formed in the city when I was surrounded by millions of people, most of whom I did not know and would never meet. I was curt and rude, and I did not consider the sensitivities of others except when I needed something from them. I assumed that I would have an unending supply of strangers to treat rudely, until I realized that I was running out of people to be insensitive to. I had only a few neighbors in the valley that was my new home, and I realized that if I wanted friends there, I needed to change my behavior.

Becoming multisensory creates a similar insight. We begin to see ourselves as long-term neighbors in eternity, and we realize that the sooner we begin treating one another with kindness, the better it will be for all. Actors who travel together in the same troupe develop an appreciation for their shared history. For example, they remember plays in which one was the hero and the other was the villain and plays in which one was the father and the other was the mother. Over time, each plays the roles of warrior, priestess, ruler and ruled, oppressor and oppressed, best friend and cruel enemy. All of them have played roles as black, red, brown, yellow, and white characters, as mothers and fathers, sisters and brothers, and explored every possible relationship through their roles. Like these actors, we are beginning to recognize one another apart from the production we are currently in.

A five-sensory individual sees her life as the only production she knows or will know. A multisensory individual sees her life as one of many in which she has appeared in the past and will appear in the future. She does not confuse fellow actors with the roles that they play—with the heroes or villains they appear to be in the moment—but as fellow travelers who, like her, are learning from each role that they play and carrying forward into future productions what they learn, and also what they do not learn.

Multisensory perception brings with it awareness of intelligence, wisdom, and compassion that are not our own any more than the humor of a friend belongs to us. We experience helping hands that cannot be seen. For example, I outlined each of the chapters of my first book, *The Dancing Wu Li Masters: An Overview of the New Physics*, before I began to write, but when I began, ideas occurred to me that were not in the outlines. Each time, I left the outline behind and wrote about the new ideas instead. Sometimes I would return to the outline and sometimes I wouldn't. One day I realized that the chapters I had written so far fit together perfectly, as though I had planned them that way. I also realized that they were more intelligent and funny than I was. Eventually, I realized that I was not writing the book alone!

All creative people—photographers, writers, musicians, architects, artists—recognize this experience. Parents recognize it when they say exactly what needs to be said to a child and what they say is appropriate, complete, and satisfying. Ancient Greeks called this experience communicating with the Muses—spirits that inspire creativity—and they called upon the Muses often. "To me and through me," they cried, "tell me the story of our people!" and from these ancient Greeks flowed the dramas and philosophies that shaped the Western world.

As we become multisensory, we can speak of the Muses in more accurate terms. They are nonphysical guides and Teachers. Imagine Friends who know everything about you—including your fears, aspirations, shame, and joy. Their only goal is to assist you in growing spiritually, and you cannot deceive or manipulate them. They are available anytime, anyplace, to answer any question. We each have such Friends, and their home is nonphysical reality.

Christians call nonphysical reality heaven and hell; Buddhists and Hindus call it the interval between lifetimes, among other things; and Aboriginal people call it the unseen world. Few, however, have experienced nonphysical reality because humanity, for the most part, has been limited to the perceptions of the five senses until recently. Now that we are becoming multisensory, faith in what lies beyond the five senses is being replaced by the experience of it.

The newly discovered enormity of the Universe, what we are, and our place in it are becoming part of our experience just as the ocean becomes part of the experience of one who discovers it for the first time. He sees clear water caress the beach and feels coolness on his feet. Shells and pebbles tumble toward him and away as waves wash in and out. He looks to the horizon, and yet even the vastness that he sees is a small part of the ocean before him. He cannot fathom its depth, know the creatures that inhabit it, or glimpse the mountains beneath its surface. Even if he swims as far from the beach as he can, he still cannot experience the scope of the ocean.

In a similar way, a larger arena of Life is becoming visible to us. Different values and goals are emerging. We are called in unexpected ways to contribute gifts that we did not know we had. Our new frontier is the nonphysical Universe of wisdom and compassion and our relationships with it and one another. No territory has been more thrilling and challenging to explore, or has held more potential for reward. This territory is the new consciousness of the new humanity. It is very different from the consciousness of the Vikings who discovered North America, from those who sailed with Columbus, and from the colonialists who exploited it. It is very different from the consciousness of all who, since the first humans, have explored the domain of the five senses in order to conquer it and use it for their gain.

This is the new land, and we are the new explorers.

2
Soul View

Mount Shasta and its adjoining summit, Shastina, rise nearly three miles above sea level and more than two miles above the valley floor where I lived for thirteen years. They dominate the land, visible for a hundred miles when weather and terrain permit. Like solitary giants they impose themselves without competition. Their beauty fascinates, their extraordinary mass quiets the mind, and their majesty is matchless. Outside of Seattle another great mountain, Mount Rainier, also dominates the land, drawing the eye, calling the heart, and incomparably defining all around it. These mountains appear to be unconnected marvels, but they are not. Mount Rainier lies at the northern end of a mountain range that extends southward hundreds of miles to California, to Mount Shasta, and beyond.

Unlike the Sierra Nevada, the Rocky Mountains, the Alps, Pyrenees, Himalayas, and Andes, this range is almost entirely underground. Only its highest summits are visible. The elevations of Mount Shasta and Mount Rainier—each over fourteen thousand feet—reveal the magnitude of this range (the Cascade Mountains) and the unseen geological dynamics that created them. In the same way, circumstances and events that appear to be unrelated to five-sensory perception are not. The nonphysical dynamics that connect and generate them, like most of the Cascade range, are invisible. Multisensory perception illuminates these dynamics and makes them useful. These "subterranean" dynamics all have to do with creation and responsibility.

The first is the Universal Law of Creation. This Law is simple. We create our experiences with our choices. All humans experience themselves as actors in a play that someone else (or no one) has written. Like stage characters following the same script without choice, they are born, live, and die. Between birth and death some improvise, some experiment, and some just survive, but they are all born and they all die. They hope for the best and brace against the worst. They celebrate good fortune and lament bad luck. This perception is created by the limitations of five-sensory perception. The five senses can detect only physical circumstances, and the intellect concludes that if physical circumstances are not connected by physical causes and physical effects, they are not connected. This is like concluding that Mount Rainier and Mount Shasta are not connected.

Five-sensory humans believe that actions create consequences. That is a small part of the story. Multisensory humans know that the intention behind an action creates the consequences of the action. An intention is a quality of consciousness. It is the reason for the action, the motivation for acting. The intention to support a friend by giving him information that he needs and does not know, for example, produces constructive consequences. The intention to prove that you are smarter than a friend produces destructive consequences. The former opens you to others. The latter closes your heart.

The second dynamic is the Universal Law of Cause and Effect. It has the same form as the physical law of cause and effect that is the foundation of empirical (five-sensory) science, namely, that every cause produces an effect and every effect has a cause. The physical law of cause and effect connects physical causes with physical effects. This enables the conscious creation of physical consequences, such as a lunar landing or a flu vaccine. As we have seen, the physical law of cause and effect is the only causal dynamic that is visible to five-sensory humans, and as a result many events and circumstances that are intimately related appear unconnected to them.

Multisensory humans see the role of nonphysical causes

(intentions) as well as physical causes (actions) in the creative process. In fact, they see that choice of intention *is* the creative process. From the multisensory perspective, the physical law of cause and effect is a reflection in the domain of time, space, matter, and duality of the Universal Law of Cause and Effect. In other words, multisensory humans are able to see why so many actions produce consequences that appear to be unintended. They are not actually unintended.

When you are aware of your intention (cause), you can predict the consequences that it will create (effect). When you are not aware of it, the experience that it creates will be surprising and painful. For example, when you intend to exploit a neighbor (and exploit him), someone in your future will exploit you. When you intend to care for another (and care for her), others in your future will care for you. The Universal Law of Cause and Effect is called the Golden Rule in the West and karma in the East. Remembering it when you choose your intentions enables you to create a loving and healthy future. Ignoring it insures that your future will bring unhealthy and painful experiences.

Remembering it also enables you to locate past intentions that you were not aware of. Each unexpected and painful experience points you back to the intention that created it, if you are looking for it. You may be surprised at how many hidden agendas (unconscious intentions) you will discover that you had (or have).

The third dynamic is the Universal Law of Attraction. Energy attracts like energy. For example, when you are angry you attract angry people and you live in an angry world. When you are greedy, you attract greedy people and you live in a greedy world. When you are loving, you attract loving people and you live in a loving world. It is that simple. Five-sensory humans believe that their world determines their beliefs. Multisensory individuals know that it validates their beliefs. If you believe that the world is dog-eat-dog, you become one of the dogs and you live in a world of dogfights. If you believe that the world is miraculous, you become a miracle and you live in a world of miraculous people. Five-sensory individuals think, "I will believe it when I see it." Multisensory individuals know, "I will see it when I believe it."

Some individuals have multisensory perception now, others are acquiring it, and all humans will be multisensory within a few generations. As we become multisensory our experiences become richer, more meaningful, and more informative. Internal processes become more significant than external circumstances. Multisensory perception redirects our attention one hundred and eighty degrees from the focus of five-sensory perception—from outside of ourselves to inside of ourselves. What is behind our eyes becomes more important to us than what is in front of them.

We experience ourselves and others as part of a larger fabric of Life, and our values shift in unexpected ways. Sometimes our perceptions surprise us, for example, when we discover that we know things about others that we have no way of knowing. For instance, we sense that a gruff individual is kind and that an individual who appears kind is not. Friends call while we are thinking about them, or tell us that we called while they were thinking of us. Everyday experiences, such as greeting a fellow passenger on the bus, become meaningful, appropriate, and gratifying.

Intuition replaces the intellect as the primary decision-making faculty. Five-sensory humans are curious about intuition at best. It is a novelty to them, if they think of it at all. From the multisensory perspective, intuition is the voice of the nonphysical world. It is direct access to nonphysical but real sources of compassion and wisdom that are beyond what we can give to one another. These are our nonphysical guides and Teachers. The nonphysical world is nonsense (literally) to five-sensory humans. It is central to the experience of millions of multisensory humans, and it is becoming central to millions more who are becoming multisensory. The new vista of multisensory perception is non-physical reality, our relationship to it, our relationships to one another in it, and our nonphysical guides and Teachers.

Multisensory perception is as different from five-sensory perception as the experiences of someone who cannot read are from those of a reader. Love poems, dissertations, histories, and stories are inaccessible to nonreaders, except through others. They see only marks on paper, meaningless lines of little interest and no value, so they cannot appreciate them or benefit from them. Five-sensory humans are (metaphorically speaking) nonreaders. Circumstances and events that are meaningful and useful to multisensory humans are meaningless and useless to them.

The physical world is the entirety of existence to five-sensory humans. Even if they do not think about it that way (for example, they believe in heaven and hell, or reincarnation), they experience it that way. Multisensory humans see the domain of the five senses—from galaxies to subatomic particles—as a part of nonphysical reality. Perceptions of the five senses do not disappear for multisensory humans. They take on new meaning.

From the five-sensory perspective we are bodies and minds in time and space, our actions create consequences, and our influence propagates through physical causes and physical effects. From the multisensory perspective we are immortal souls as well as personalities, the larger part of us exists in nonphysical reality, our intentions create our experiences, and our influence extends far beyond what we can see, hear, taste, touch, and smell.

From the perspective of the five senses, "bad things happen to good people" and "good things happen to bad people." From the multisensory perspective, appropriate things happen to all people, everywhere, all the time. Multisensory perception makes the concepts of "chance," "random," "accidental," and "fate" meaningless. Choices made in anger create painful consequences; choices made in love create loving consequences. If you plant corn, corn grows. If you plant tomatoes, you harvest tomatoes. An individual who does not understand why his life is painful instead of joyful is like a farmer who does not understand why barley is growing in his field instead of lettuce. He is not aware of the seeds that he has planted, or when, or how. Multisensory perception allows you to become aware of the seeds you are planting (your intentions) so that you can know in advance what crop you will harvest (the consequences of your intentions).

A five-sensory human sees her life as a book with a beginning, middle, and end. A multisensory human sees her life as a chapter in a book of many chapters. She knows that some of her experiences result from what happened in earlier chapters and that her decisions determine some of the things that will happen in later chapters.

Five-sensory perception is like looking through a window. You are not part of what you see. Multisensory perception is like looking into a mirror. You see yourself and ways to change yourself constructively. As five-sensory humans become multisensory they are attracted to new goals. Cooperation becomes more attractive than competition. Sharing becomes more attractive than hoarding. Harmony becomes more attractive than discord. Reverence becomes more attractive than exploitation. As you begin to travel toward these goals, the reflection in the mirror changes. For example, when you hoard, the Universal Law of Cause and Effect insures that you will experience the pain of needing and not having what others could give to you if they chose. When you share, it insures that you will experience the support of others who share with you because they choose to.

The entire human experience is in transition. Old goals are falling away and old victories no longer satisfy. New winds are blowing, new songs are calling to be sung, and new understandings are blooming. Sometimes strong and clear, sometimes subtle and fleeting, multisensory perceptions are appearing in millions of humans—the initial stage of a transformation that is profoundly altering the human experience. This transformation is occurring regardless of our choices, but what we do with it is a different matter.

Multisensory perception will not make us kind, patient, caring, considerate, reverent, or loving. It makes us more aware. We see more than the five senses can show us, but we must decide how to use our expanded awareness. Five-sensory humans change circumstances or wait for others to change them. Multisensory humans change themselves. Multisensory perception illuminates the path to personal mastery and requires a decision, moment by moment, to walk it or not, to cause healthy or unhealthy effects, to create constructive or destructive consequences. The new vista of multisensory perception makes our creative power impossible to ignore and our choices impossible to avoid. It transforms the experiences of a life into a continual series of learning opportunities that unfold in a full-color, surround-sound, always-up-to-the-moment educational environment with billions of students, each with a custom-tailored curriculum. This is the Earth school.

Multisensory perception illuminates the nonphysical causes of endless conflict; hunger, starvation, and poverty; pervasive brutality and exploitation; the spread of violence and destruction despite every violent and destructive effort to contain them; the unrepentant rapaciousness of capitalism; the brutal imposition of one religion upon another; and murder in the name of the divine, to name a few. As a result, ways to change these things also become available to us.

Five-sensory humans see their lives as unexplainable except in terms of the five senses, just as five-sensory scientists see consciousness as inexplicable in an inert (dead) Universe. Multisensory humans see their lives as a continual flow of gifts from the Universe—gifts of relevant symbolism and potential for spiritual growth. Five-sensory individuals think their lives have no purpose except what they ascribe to them or what others have told

them. To multisensory humans no experience is without purpose, meaning, and opportunity to grow spiritually. Five-sensory
humans see a human birth as a physical event. Multisensory
humans see it as a dramatic act of spiritual responsibility, the
voluntary incarnation of an immortal soul.

Multisensory perceptions provide access to the perspective
of the soul. They are not the experiences of the soul, but they
reveal our lives as ongoing encounters with appropriate-at-each-
moment, always-up-to-date experiences that are perfect for the
spiritual growth of each individual involved, given the choices
that he or she has made.

The soul view does not heal your pain. It places the healing
of it squarely and irrevocably in the context of spiritual development.

3
The Ultimate Pain

*L*ove is the most misunderstood and abused word in our vocabulary. Love is now the engine of our evolution, but in a way that is very surprising and disturbing. The evolution of multisensory humanity requires learning to love, exploring every aspect of love, and enjoying every possibility of love. The only way that we can now evolve, therefore, is elegantly simple: discover, experience, and heal the parts of ourselves that do not love, and discover, experience, and cultivate the parts that do.

"Unconditional love" is redundant, like "wet water." Love includes. Conditions exclude. In joy and pain, success and failure, health and illness, youth and old age—Love is. Love cannot be disappointed because it has no expectations. Love, Universe, Consciousness, and Light are the same. The Universe is everything—stars and the vastness of space, cells in bodies and sidewalks by streets, seeds, soil, all of us and more. Everything is a form of Life, of Consciousness, of Light, of Love. Therefore, it is impossible to be unloved. It is also impossible not to belong—not be part of the Universe of Light, of Love, of Consciousness—and yet the deepest pain of every human is needing to be loved and feeling unlovable, longing to love and feeling incapable of loving, wanting to belong and feeling unworthy.

Learning to love brings you with relentless compassion into intimate contact with parts of your personality that do not love, do not want to love, and do not care about love. These are the parts that you need to heal. They seek revenge, judge, criticize, blame, and more. Love forgives and accepts all—the kind and the cruel, the selfish and the selfless, the loving and the unloving.

"Unconditional love" confuses need with love. Love is blissful and requires nothing. Need is painful, has conditions, and always demands more. For example, when you buy a new car (house, suit, bicycle) that you have been longing to own, your need for the car (painful) is replaced by your need to protect it (painful). When you create a relationship, at last, that gives you the security, sex, or family that you dreamed of, your fear of not finding such a relationship (painful) is replaced by your fear of losing it (painful). These are not experiences of love. They are experiences of need. They may look and feel like love to the one who needs, but the experience of attachment always reveals otherwise. The experience of attachment *is* the experience of need.

"Unrequited love" is unrequited need in disguise—experiences of one human reaching futilely for fulfillment through another, withering in loneliness, or drowning in despair. Painful experiences are not love no matter how much they appear to be. For example, a friend of mine raised a small dog from a puppy, looked forward to seeing it every evening, and played with it on weekends. The dog was a big part of his life. One afternoon it ran away. He called, whistled, and searched. Family and friends came to help. Suddenly in the midst of communal whistling and calling it reappeared, carefree as before. My friend rushed toward it with anger distorting his face. The dog cowered, too frightened to run. It whined once as he swept it off its feet and shook it in the air. He furiously shouted at the terrified animal not to run away again. When his family tried to calm him he shouted at them, "It's my dog, dammit!"

Later, embarrassed but unrepentant, he explained, "I love that dog. I love it as much as anyone in my family. That is why I was angry when it ran away and why I needed to make it understand not to run away again." He mistook need for love. One part of his personality loved the dog, but another part *needed* the dog and was terrified to lose it. That part became active when the dog ran away.

Need requires a return on investment, whether the investment is time, money, or "love." The dog did not provide the return that a frightened part of my friend's personality expected. He did not think about investments or returns but a frightened part of his personality that he was unaware of did, and it became furious when the animal ran away. Beneath his fury was fear of losing something important. He thought that was his dog, but it was not. It was what the dog brought him, at least temporarily—experiences of feeling loved and lovable, belonging, and being a part of Life.

The search for value and self-worth is always desperate because the pain of wanting to be loved and feeling unlovable, wanting to love and feeling incapable of loving, needing to belong and feeling excluded is unbearable. This is the pain of powerlessness. It lies at the core of the human experience. Powerlessness is the experience of feeling intrinsically defective, inherently ugly, and without value. It is the fear that if others could see you as you really are, they would not want to be with you. It is self-hatred. At bottom, it is the experience of not being worthy of your life. Nothing is more excruciating.

Even if you do not recognize the pain of powerlessness, you may be surprised to discover it in yourself anyway. If you look beneath your experiences, especially when you are angry, jealous, resentful, etc., or immersed in other painful emotions that are so familiar you think they are "just who I am," you will find deeper layers of painful experiences, each capable of providing you helpful information about yourself. The bottom layer is always the pain of powerlessness. Beneath the anger of my friend when his dog ran away, for example, was the need for his dog; beneath that lay his need to control the dog; and beneath that was his need for the world to be the way that he wants it to be (which the dog ignored). Each layer temporarily masks the pain of powerlessness.

We always feel the pain of powerlessness when the world is not the way we want it to be, for example, a spouse leaves, a child dies, we lose a job, or feel betrayed. To mask it we become angry, jealous, vengeful, depressed, withdrawn, and so on. We do not think in terms of powerlessness or pain. Instead we explode in anger and blame the circumstance (the way my friend became angry and blamed his dog), withdraw emotionally, become tearful, seek revenge, or overeat, overwork, watch pornography, use drugs, drink, gamble, and so on, always seeing circumstances (including people) as the cause of our painful experiences and destructive behaviors. All we can see are external circumstances, and we are at the mercy of them.

Avoiding the pain of powerlessness continually determines our perceptions, intentions, and actions. We use people and things to make us feel valuable, worthy, complete, and whole, for example, a spouse, a child, or a job. Whatever you use, it is very important to your sense of security and value. Some people use fame, others use wealth, others use their education, and yet others use their intelligence, humor, house, or political opinion. When you use anything to influence (manipulate and control) others in order to feel safe and valuable, you are avoiding the pain of powerlessness.

To say that humanity is insecure is to state the obvious. How we respond to the pain of powerlessness is the difference between human evolution before the appearance of multisensory perception and after it (now). Five-sensory humans avoid the pain of powerlessness by controlling and manipulating circumstances, including people. When a child dies, for example, they conceive another; when a business fails, they build another; when a relationship falls apart, they find another partner. They choose clothing, cars, and hairstyles to make themselves feel attractive, competent, or sexual. They are proud of their strength, intelligence, beauty, education, wealth, fame, home, or skis—anything that makes them feel valuable and safe. They dominate, please, rebel, shop, overeat, smoke, drink, and more in order to manipulate and control in order to feel valuable and safe. The wealthiest of us and the most impoverished share the pain of powerlessness. All flee it by attempting to manipulate and control circumstances. This is the pursuit of external power.

Trying to keep external power is like trying to store water in a paper sack. It can be gained and lost, inherited and stolen, earned and destroyed. For example, elections are won (more ability to manipulate and control) and lost (less ability to manipulate and control); stock portfolios go up in value (more ability to manipulate and control) and down (less ability to manipulate and control); strong bodies (more ability to manipulate and control) become weak (less ability to manipulate and control); and quick minds (more ability to manipulate and control) deteriorate (less ability to manipulate and control). One style goes out of favor (less ability to manipulate and control with it) and another comes into favor (more ability to manipulate and control with it), and so on.

Human history—individual and collective—is a chronicle of the pursuit of external power. Writ large or small, the story is the same—safety and comfort in the ability to manipulate and control, danger and distress in the absence of it, and competition to obtain it. The pursuit of external power is not limited to the young or the old, wealthy or indigent, urban or rural, educated or illiterate. It is the pursuit of all humans because the need to belong, feel safe, be loved, and be worthy is shared by all. Once you recognize external power you will see it everywhere. Cultures, religions, and nations pursue it. Businesses, cities, and neighborhoods pursue it. Siblings, spouses, and parents fight for the same reasons that corporations fight—they want to control one another.

Death is the ultimate failure of external power and, therefore, the most terrifying of all five-sensory experiences. The quest for external power is a story without end, the black hole of the human experience, the perpetual expression of perpetual insecurity.

No one noticed or explored the nature and origin of external power before because prior to the emergence of multisensory perception no other understanding of power existed. External power and five-sensory humanity are inseparable. External power enabled five-sensory humanity to survive. Now the pursuit of it creates only violence and destruction. This is a very big change. What was once good medicine has become toxic.

The potential of five-sensory humanity was a world without physical need—a world in which all are sheltered, clothed, fed, and healthy. That potential has gone unfulfilled and the time for fulfilling it has run out. Five-sensory humanity is coming to an end. It could have created physical paradise for all, but it did not. In addition to its constructive accomplishments, it also created ecological devastation, horrifying weapons, caste systems, genocide, and global exploitation. If five-sensory humanity had pursued external power with reverence, its short history and relationship with the Earth would have been very different.

During my first event with Native American youth I met an elder who touched me deeply. I had never seen lightness and groundedness, humor and wisdom, compassion and clarity combined so seamlessly. He was as nimble as a young man, but he had seen more than seventy winters. He was Indian and cowboy in one—a chief who wore a Stetson hat and a Cutting Horse Championship belt buckle. Before the end of the event, he adopted me as his nephew. We grew closer and closer until he passed on a decade later. I treasured him, his family, and our relationship. Once he told me, "Buffalo calves are always at the center of the herd where they are safest. The old buffalos travel on the outside of the herd where they give themselves to their brothers, the wolves." Then he said after a pause, "Nephew, I am becoming like those old buffalos. My life is all for the people now." He meant all people.

Native wisdom honors external power with reverence, but the pursuit of external power without reverence has destroyed most Native cultures. Christ taught his disciples to love others more than their own lives, but the pursuit of external power without reverence has deformed his teaching into a fantasy goal. This story is long and repetitive. External power without reverence has turned the human experience brutal. Millions of individuals wish that they had not been born, and millions more long to die. The usefulness of external power—with or without reverence—has come to an end, just as five-sensory humanity has come to an end.

Multisensory humanity has begun. Multisensory humans see what five-sensory humans cannot—that each pursuit of external power is a flight from the pain of powerlessness. They can respond differently to the pain of powerlessness because they can see a different kind of power.

4

The Butterfly Effect

You are not as invisible or powerless as you think. You do not need to create wealth, recognition, admiration, or praise to influence the world around you. Your impact on the world is significant whether or not you are aware of it, and even whether or not you desire it. In the early 1960s a research meteorologist at MIT who had created a computer program to model the weather was in a hurry to reprint the results of a simulation he had already run. To speed the process, he entered only the first three digits of the original six that he had used to define each initial condition in the simulation (for example, he rounded off ".506127" to ".506"). When the printout arrived, it was entirely different from the original. At first he thought his computer had malfunctioned; then he remembered his changes. He did not suspect that such minor variances could affect the results, much less change them dramatically, but he was mistaken. His changes made a *huge* difference. In fact, the computer predicted entirely different weather conditions.

This sensitive dependence on initial conditions has come to be called the *butterfly effect* because the large magnitude of the change in predicted weather in relation to the minute variances in initial conditions is poetically analogous to a butterfly changing the weather on the other side of the world by moving its wings. The butterfly effect is a helpful metaphor for your enormous creative capacity. Most people think of themselves as without influence except in their immediate circumstances, and even there they often feel powerless. "If I had money," they think, or "If I were an actor, a billionaire, a sports hero, gorgeous, brilliant, a professor, or an executive, I would have influence. If I had a yacht, or a mountain bike, or the shoes I saw on sale, people would listen when I speak, or at least some of them would notice me." (This is the pursuit of external power.)

Your decisions are continually creating new "initial conditions," and the weather that those varying conditions are continually changing is your experience. Small decisions in the moment turn out to be not so small in retrospect. Saying yes instead of no changes your experience. Pushing people away instead of inviting them to come close changes your experience, even if you do not make that choice consciously. Acting in anger, for example, even when you feel righteous or justified, pushes people away. Then you are lonely because your anger pushed people away. Then you become angry again, and again push people away without thinking about what acting on your anger is creating. It is making big changes in the weather.

Judging people also pushes them away, even if you do not express your judgments. You may judge someone as incompetent, for example, or unattractive, inept, or self-centered, and your judgment will push him away whether or not you express it. You may address him politely, smile, or express false appreciation, but he will feel your judgment. He may not realize that you are pushing him away, but he will feel a disconnect between your display of appreciation and his experience of not being appreciated. He may simply find himself avoiding you when he can. Your concern for the well-being of others will attract them to you whether or not you express it (Universal Law of Attraction). When you act in their behalf, they feel supported or comforted, even if you do not smile or ingratiate yourself. You, also, can sense when someone who appears gruff is kind, and when someone who appears kind is not to be trusted. These are multisensory perceptions.

Once I was camping on a moonless night. When darkness engulfed the forest, leaving my tent became hazardous. Small stones, easy to turn an ankle on, larger boulders, easy to smash a toe into, and fallen branches, easy to trip over, lay around it. When dawn arrived (or I turned on a flashlight), stepping over or around them became easy. Multisensory perception is the dawn (and we didn't have flashlights before it arrived). Now you can use your intuition to help you. For example, a friend of mine was rushing to leave Taiwan before the full force of a typhoon enveloped the island. Standing in line at the airport to check in, he had a premonition not to fly, but he was so close to boarding, and the typhoon was building in strength. He checked his bags and boarded. In the driving rain and raging wind, the pilot mistook a closed runway for the active runway, and as the huge airliner lifted off the ground it crashed into a crane, ripping off a wing and igniting a fire that killed most of the passengers. It took years of surgery, therapy, and struggles with pain before my friend began to regain his life. He knew not to board the plane, but he disregarded what he knew.

You have probably had similar experiences. If you have a hunch to remain at home, for example, and then leave anyway and slip on ice, you will regret not paying attention to your hunch just as my friend regretted not paying attention to his. Looking out the window (five-sensory perception) will show you ice outside, but not that you are more likely to slip on it today. Everyone has had the experience of saying, "I *knew* I shouldn't have done that!" or "I *knew* I should have done that!" No empirical (five-sensory) preflight investigation could have revealed that the pilot was more likely to mistake a runway under construction for an active runway on that particular stormy night—only that the probability for error was increased. In the same way, no predeparture investigation could have revealed that you were more likely to slip on ice that day than on other icy days, only that the probability of a slip was increased. However, these are not issues of probability. My friend *knew* that he shouldn't board, and you have probably had the experience of *knowing* that you should not do what you were considering, and done it anyway.

If you have a hunch, for example, not to bring up a certain subject with a friend because it will cause reactions in her (such as anger, jealousy, or fear), and you bring it up anyway and ruin the opportunity to cocreate with her that day, you *know* that you could have avoided those consequences. This is another way of saying that you know you could have created differently. You could have chosen differently, and different consequences would have followed. If my friend had chosen differently at the Taiwan airport he would still be enjoying the athletic, pain-free body that he had.

Multisensory perception puts the butterfly effect, your choices, and your creative power into a new context. Instead of experiencing yourself as an insignificant, invisible, powerless individual struggling with a random or cruel world, you become aware of a different possibility: You are a powerful, creative, compassionate, and loving spirit acting like an insignificant, invisible, powerless individual and, in the process, creating painful consequences with your anger, jealousy, rage, fear, and vengefulness. Your need to please or dominate, experiences of superiority or inferiority, and obsessive, compulsive, and addictive behaviors prevent you from this larger and healthier experience of yourself and create even more painful experiences. Your choices do not go unnoticed any more than the movement of the butterfly's wings went unnoticed, so to speak. On the other side of the world a sunny day turned gray, or a violent storm calmed.

The butterfly effect refers to the influence of physical causes (small-scale) on physical phenomena (large-scale) and illustrates the dramatic importance of "initial conditions" that are so small that they can easily be overlooked. Multisensory perception expands awareness beyond physical causes to nonphysical causes as well. It reveals new realms to explore and use. For example, it allows you to experiment with the nonphysical "initial conditions" in your life that are so easy to overlook you may not have even considered them but that are actually of huge importance.

These are your intentions. Your intentions determine your experiences whether or not you are aware of them. When you are not aware of them, the consequences they create will surprise you, and they will be painful.

Intention means different things to five-sensory individuals than it does to multisensory individuals. Five-sensory individuals think of intentions in terms such as "to get a new job." Multisensory individuals go deeper. They ask, "Why do I intend to get a new job?" One reason might be, for example, "to make more money" (other reasons might be to have more prestige, work closer to home, or have a greater sense of meaning), and they keep asking until they find their real reason. Their quest for the deepest Why leads them to their actual intention. For example, a parent may intend to make more money in order to send her child to college. Beneath this intention lie deeper intentions. One parent may intend to send her child to college because she feels obligated, her family expects it, or her neighbor's children are going to college. Another may intend to expose her child to languages, cultures, and disciplines that will stimulate her creativity and passion. These are different intentions, and they will create different consequences.

The Why beneath the Why (and sometimes the Why beneath that, etc.) is the intention that creates consequences. That is the Why that determines the experiences of your life. The parent who sends her child to college to make her (the parent) feel better about herself, as good as her neighbors, or to avoid family disapproval is concerned about herself. The parent who supports her child with the gift of education is concerned about her child. One is taking and the other is giving. One is motivated by fear, and the other is motivated by love. Both parents set into motion the Universal Law of Cause and Effect and the Universal Law of Attraction and, therefore, create different consequences with their different intentions. The first parent will experience the pain of discovering that someone she loves is using her for his or her own well-being (Universal Law of Cause and Effect) and will attract to her people with hidden agendas (Universal Law of Attraction). The second parent will experience the joy of being cared for without conditions (Universal Law of Cause and Effect) and will draw to herself people who are concerned for her (Universal Law of Attraction).

To five-sensory perception, these actions are identical—a parent sends a child to college. Without knowing the intention beneath the action, however, it is not possible to know the consequences that the action will create. When I first learned to ski, I would carry my skis on my shoulder with the short ends in front of me and the long ends with the tips behind. However, I soon learned how dangerous that was because I kept forgetting how far the tips extended. When I turned, they swung around fast, causing people to duck and lunge out of the way (and complain). Not knowing your intentions is like carrying long skis on your shoulder into a china shop. Every time you turn, something behind you breaks and you can't see what caused the damage, but you are responsible for it.

Using your creative power without knowing your intentions is like driving a car with the windshield painted black. You travel, but you do not know where. You expect to arrive at a destination, but when you get out of the car (or the car crashes into something), you discover that where you thought you were going and where you went are different. If you have a need to please people, for example, you will be surprised (and probably have been many times) to discover that they eventually push you away. When your intention is to see a smile or be appreciated in order to feel safe and valuable (this is the pursuit of external power), you will always feel the pain of rejection when you see a frown instead or your efforts are not appreciated. Eventually (or immediately) you will feel abused. Your compulsive efforts to please have a price, and when it is not paid, you become angry. You expect to arrive at appreciation, but you arrive instead at rejection and anger—a very different destination.

Most people drive with the windshield painted black, for example, the husband who provides his wife with home and security and then becomes angry when she does not provide him comfort and sex on demand. Like my friend who thought he loved his dog but became enraged when it failed to meet his expectations (hidden agendas), the husband reached a different destination (frustration, anger, and pain) than the one he antici-pated (domestic bliss). If you think your windshield is clear, ask yourself how many times you have felt angry, or at least miffed, when someone dismissed a gift that you gave, or threw it away. ("Another sweater? I've got one already and you know I don't like brown.") Those experiences always signal the presence of an intention that you were not aware of, one that is different from the intention you thought you held.

There is a common misconception that the healthiest inten-tion is to "feel good." The addict in an alley injects heroin because it makes him feel good, but it is not making him healthy or even getting him out of the alley. On the other hand, the alcoholic who has just stopped drinking is in excruciating pain, but he is becoming healthy. The healthy intention is never to pursue exter-nal power. Intending to get attention, for example, with a fast or opulent car, gorgeous spouse, beautiful home, expensive jewelry, ideal life (or anything else) because you feel inadequate, invis-ible, and powerless without it will not take you where you want to go when your destination is a life of more meaning and less emp-tiness, more joy and less pain, more love and less fear.

That life is the potential, and also the evolutionary require-ment, of multisensory humans, and all humans are becoming multisensory or soon will be. The causal connections between us are more than physical. We influence one another and all of Life with our choices of intention, and with our choices of intention we transform our experiences from fear to love (or not), and our world from brutal to compassionate (or not). We are each ultimately responsible for the well-being of all that is. The pursuit of external power is the set of initial conditions that always creates harsh weather. The more we think of ourselves as invisible or powerless, the more we wield our creative power irresponsibly (and create painful consequences). The more we blame others for our experiences, envy them, or rage at them or ourselves, the more painful consequences we create. The emergence of multisensory perception is a dawn unlike any before, and the rising sun is illuminating a new set of initial conditions that always and everywhere creates the best of all weather.

5
The Cave

The most famous philosopher of Western civilization is probably Plato (428?–347 BC). Historians generally agree that he is the most influential. He was a student of Socrates and the teacher of Aristotle. Together, these are the Big Three of Western philosophy. (*Philosophy* means "love of wisdom.") Plato wrote numerous dialogues (he adopted this way of teaching from Socrates), but my favorite is the one with his story of the cave. Individuals deep in a cave are chained in such a way that they can see only shadows on the wall of the cave. The shadows are cast by models or statues that are moved in front of a bright fire. One day a person breaks free and escapes from the cave. Standing in the sunlight for the first time, he sees the real world—not the world of shadows—and returns to tell the others what he has discovered: All that you see here are shadows! They are not real. The real world is waiting for you outside this cave if you are willing to get out of it.

Perhaps Plato was the one who broke free and returned to tell us about the real world. In any case, he is clear that we can break free also, and that the sun and the real world are waiting for us, too. They are always waiting for us. If we speak in terms of love and fear, fear is the darkness and love is the light. I do not know if Plato would have used these words, but I think that he might have agreed. Fear is a prison (cave), and love is freedom from it (the world outside). Throughout five-sensory history (which is all of human history until recently) a few multisensory humans have spoken, written, and shared about the world outside the cave—experiences of light, love, and freedom. Also, our largest religions share this message in one way or another, although they disagree on how to get out of the cave. (These disagreements keep many people in the cave.) Plato considered the world outside to be the world of perfect forms, and disciplined intellectual inquiry to be the way out of the cave.

The hero who left the cave did not walk out of it the same way that a customer in a restaurant leaves after his meal. He was chained. If leaving the cave were easy, others would have left. Only one prisoner had the intention and the courage to break free. If Plato's story speaks to you—if you long for a larger, brighter, freer, and more meaningful world—it is because you also are chained or you would have escaped to that world long ago. Plato's hero had metal around his body. Where is the metal around your body? What chains hold you so firmly that you cannot escape your familiar experiences (and, perhaps until you read Plato's allegory, did not consider the possibility of a larger, freer, and brighter world)?

How would you break free if you could not see your chains but you could see the consequences of them? For example, suppose you discovered that every time someone speaks to you impolitely, you become offended, or feel belittled. You connect the dots between your most recent experience of belittlement and the one before that, and the one before that, as far back as you can remember. In each case, the person who offended you was different, but your experience was the same. You are imprisoned in a repeating experience, chained in such a way that you can see only it again and again, but where are your chains?

Imagine becoming angry, impatient, vengeful, rejected, or jealous not once, but again and again. Everyone has painful experiences that repeat without end, such as remorse, guilt, resentment, overwhelm, and feelings of inadequacy, to name a few. Each time one occurs, you think that you can stop it by changing the person or circumstance that caused it. For example, you divorce the spouse that you think causes your anger, leave the job that you think causes your anger, move out of the neighborhood, country, or family that you think causes your anger, but no matter how many times you change something or someone that you think causes your anger, your anger returns (or doesn't leave). You are imprisoned in anger, but where are your chains? You live in a painful world—friends are angry, colleagues are angry, you are angry—but you cannot leave.

Imagine that every time someone offers you sex, you cannot refuse, no matter how destructive the consequences might be. You could become infected with AIDS, infect someone you love with AIDS, or destroy your marriage, but those things do not matter to you in the moment. You are chained to the need for sex. Imagine that every time you see ice cream, a colleague offers dessert, or you join friends who are snacking, you eat and you feel powerless to stop; or that every time someone offers you a drink, a drug, or a cigarette, you cannot resist. Some people live their lives in regret, jealousy, inferiority, superiority, anger, fear, resentment, or overwhelm, even when they want to change. There are as many prisons as there are painful emotions, obsessions, compulsions, and addictions.

The five senses cannot detect your chains, but multisensory perception operates independently of the five senses. A five-sensory exploration of anger, for example, can track hormone levels, respiratory and circulatory rates, and a variety of physiological correlates to anger, but it cannot locate chains. An intellectual inquiry connects past and current experiences of anger, catalogues similarities and differences and thoughts that precede and follow them, but it cannot locate chains, either. Multisensory perception makes your chains visible, but in a surprising way. You *feel* them.

They do not reveal themselves by the touch of metal on flesh, but by physical sensations in certain areas of your body that appear under certain conditions. Multisensory perception allows you to become a detective, always looking for information about your chains. Eventually, you will assemble a picture of them. For example, you may feel a sharp pain and a tightening in your chest, a pressure on your forehead, and a dull burning in your stomach. That is an experience of a chain. Sometimes the pain in your chest is dull instead of sharp, your stomach flutters instead of burns, and your throat contracts. That is the experience of another chain. Sometimes sensations are pleasant. Sometimes they are painful in one area and pleasant in others. The more you notice these sensations, especially when you are upset, the more familiar you become with a continually changing interior landscape that is unique to you.

Different circumstances create different sensations, and because your circumstances are always changing, the sensations in your body are always changing, too. For example, imagine that you see a dear friend from your childhood in a café. Your heart opens, and you begin to smile. You walk toward her, eager to reconnect. If you were paying attention to the sensations in your body, you would feel wonderful sensations. Your chest, throat, and solar plexus (midtrunk) areas, for example, would feel relaxed, warm, and open. Imagine that when you return home you find a letter from the audit division of the Internal Revenue Service. If you were paying attention to your sensations, you would notice how very different they are from the sensations that you experienced when you saw your friend. The IRS letter and the encounter with your friend are both surprises, but the sensations they produce in you are quite different.

It is easy to distinguish between painful and pleasant sensations (if you know how to monitor your interior landscape), and to recognize your chains (they hurt). At first painful sensations appear to be caused by circumstances, for example, receiving notice of the audit, but after a while you will make a very important discovery (one of the most important in your life): Your painful sensations recur, but the apparent causes of them frequently change. The same painful sensations that tormented you in your former marriage, job, or city repeat wherever you are and whomever you are with. Each time they do, you react in the same way that you did the last time, for example, you become angry, jealous, frightened, vengeful, or overwhelmed. If you habitually shout when you become angry, you will shout again. If you habitually withdraw, you will withdraw again, and so on. In other words, your behavior is predictable. You do again the same thing that you did the last time you became angry (or jealous, vengeful, or frightened, etc.). You are in a prison.

Some people are imprisoned by anger, some by jealousy, and some by vengefulness, among others. Most are inmates in several prisons. They are frequently out on parole (not angry, jealous, etc., in the moment), but that does not last and they wind up in prison again. Recidivism (inmates returning to prison after getting out) is very high. Most people spend their entire lives in prisons, and they die in them—still angry, jealous, and more. They live unexamined lives (Plato's term)—chained deep in a cave where only shadows are visible. When you blame a spouse, friend, coworker, boss, or the Universe for your anger, jealousy, or any other painful experience, you are chained in a cave. Your anger, jealousy, vengefulness, fear, and other painful emotions are your chains, but blaming others or circumstances for them is no more helpful than shouting at the shadows or withdrawing from them because you do not like the way they appear or move. Your chains remain in place. While you focus on shadows, you cannot see your chains, and you cannot change what you cannot see.

People and circumstances trigger your anger, jealousy, and fear, but changing those experiences requires turning your attention toward what has been triggered (the painful experiences of your chains) and away from what triggered it (the shadows). Looking inward when you become upset (feeling the sensations in your body) instead of looking outward (attempting to change people or circumstances) allows you to explore what has been activated inside you. Until you change *that,* you will not change. You will continue to shout, weep, and withdraw as well as demand apologies, feel rejected, feel superior, feel inferior, and engage in all the destructive behaviors that you have perfected. Once you become familiar with your chains, you will know exactly what you need to change.

Strange as it sounds, prisons such as anger and jealousy are often attractive in the moment. When I gave my first workshop in San Quentin, one of the corrections officers, a bitter middle-aged woman, said, disdainfully nodding her head toward a group of inmates, "All they want is two hots and a cot." By her assessment, they could not survive on the outside, and returning to prison was a refuge for them that she resented providing. The inmates I met were genuinely terrified by San Quentin, yet statistically many of them would indeed return. The reasons were many—gravitational pull of old habits, society's distrust of ex-cons, inability to find a job, rejection—but return they did to the familiar and structured, although terrifying, environment of San Quentin.

It is less painful to become angry (jealous, vengeful, over-whelmed, etc.) than it is to feel the sensations in your body when you hate yourself, see yourself as incurably defective, unlovable, unable to love, and forever excluded from life, love, and human-ity. In other words, it is less painful in the moment to become angry, jealous, or vengeful, or to feel inferior and need to please, or superior and entitled, or to overeat, drink, or gamble than it is to experience the pain of powerlessness. Immersing yourself in anger, jealousy, or vengefulness is a refuge from this core expe-rience, and acting in anger, jealousy, or vengefulness takes you even further from it. You flee from the pain of powerlessness into a prison that shelters you from it momentarily, and then into uncontrollable actions that imprison you even more firmly.

Experiencing the pain of powerlessness directly—the painful sensations in your body that lie beneath your destructive episodes of anger, vengefulness, righteousness, and callousness—goes directly to the source of these experiences. When you have the courage and skill to experience directly the core pain that you have been running from all your life, that has generated every destructive consequence that you have created for yourself, there is no more bogeyman left to frighten you.* Then your life becomes a matter of the choices that you will make with your new awareness. If you were no longer controlled by the need to flee from the excruciating pain of self-disgust, self-loathing, and despair that has tormented you from birth, what would you choose? This is the question that you were born to ask and to answer. It is the ongoing holy inquiry that will fill your life as you begin to find your way out of the cave and into the sunlight.

Breaking your chains requires breaking old habits, abandoning old judgments about yourself and others, and experimenting with different intentions and behaviors. It requires looking at your anger, fear, jealousy, rage, and so on as dynamics that become activated in you under certain circumstances and that you can change, instead of assuming that you are intrinsically angry, jealous, etc., and will always remain that way. It requires the courage to experience all that you are feeling, moment by moment. You do not need to be imprisoned in anger or any other difficult emotion when certain circumstances occur. You can break your chains and leave.

Plato's hero did that. He left the cave, the fire, and the shadows behind. Each time you respond (choose consciously) instead of reacting (shouting, weeping, withdrawing, eating, gambling, etc.) *while you are experiencing the painful sensations in your body,*

---

* To develop this skill (experiencing your interior "chains"), I recommend you study *The Heart of the Soul: Emotional Awareness,* by my spiritual partner Linda Francis and me (Simon & Schuster, 2001). It explains emotional awareness *experientially* and helps you create it step-by-step. (Be sure to do the exercises. If you read only the text between them, you will know a lot about emotional awareness when you finish the book, but you will not be emotionally aware, and that will not help you.)

a chain weakens. When you choose again to respond instead of react, to create constructively instead of destructively, to choose consequences you are willing to assume responsibility for bringing into your life, to create health and joy instead of pain and dysfunction, it weakens further. Eventually, it will break. Sooner or later you will break all of your chains this way—choice by choice.

That is how to escape from the cave.

6

Learning to Coach

Imagine that you are the coach of a team in a game called "Life." You have numerous players, but only one of them can play at a time. The player that is on the court at the moment is always the one that represents you. Whatever that player does, it is as though you did it. If that player is elegant and graceful, you appear elegant and graceful. If that player is crude and selfish, you appear crude and selfish. Each of your players is world-class. One is an expert at anger. Everything that happens angers her, and she is continually shouting, withdrawing, and blaming someone for something. She needs no warm-up. She is always ready to play at any moment, and whenever you call upon her, she brings her top-flight anger onto the court. Another is jealous, and another seeks revenge. Your team roster is large. Another player is patient, and nothing can distract him from his patience. No matter what, when you call him he brings limitless patience to the court. Another is grateful. Whatever occurs, she is grateful for it. Another is content, another is caring, and others are kind, disdainful, impatient, overwhelmed, and anxious. Whenever you want to play contentment, caring, kindness, disdain, impatience, overwhelm, or anxiety, you can call upon them and know that they will bring that to the game flawlessly.

Your responsibility is to choose the player that you will put on the court at each moment. You can confer with others, but only you can make the final decision, and whatever you choose, you are responsible for the consequences. If you choose to play anger, you experience the consequences of anger; if you choose to play kindness, you experience the consequences of kindness;

and so on. The consequences that your players create when they play are always significant, because each is the best at what she does. You are always fielding the best jealousy, kindness, disdain, patience, vengefulness, or gratitude that you have. The court is never empty. One player is always on it, playing full out. All of your players are eager to play.

Your players will always do their very best, so when you play anger, for example, it will create the best consequences of anger possible—isolation, loneliness, shallow relationships, etc. You cannot stop experiencing the consequences that your players create for you, because one of them is always on the court. However, the more closely you watch your players and notice what experiences they create, the more skill as a coach you develop. At first, for example, playing anger might be your favorite choice, but after a while—sometimes a long while—you begin to experiment with playing patience, or jealousy, or disdain, or gratitude, all the while noting the experiences that your choices create.

Everyone around you is also a coach. Like you, they are continually choosing which of their players to put on the court. Their players never appear on your court, and your players never appear on theirs. You see the players that they choose and they see the players that you choose, but the players that they choose go onto their courts and the players that you choose go onto yours. For example, a coach near you may play anger. This will be especially exciting to some of your players. The anger, resentment, and superiority on your bench will be eager to play and will present themselves to you as strongly as they can.

Until now we have assumed that you know all the players on your team, but incredibly, many coaches do not. Most know some of their players but not all of them. The players that you know about are always waiting for your call. Those that you do not know about will take advantage of your lack of awareness and step onto the court when they please. It is as though you temporarily become unaware of the game (this is called unconsciousness) but the game, nonetheless, continues. It is always going on whether or not you are aware of it. One of your players is always on the court, always playing his or her best, and always creating consequences for you.

That is why some people become angry so often, or jealous, or hold grudges, judge others or themselves, gossip, etc. They are not yet accomplished coaches. They are not aware when certain of their players enter the game. For example, when another coach chooses to play anger (or is not aware that her anger has stepped onto her court), your anger (if you are not aware of it) will step onto your court and begin to play. If contentment was playing when this happens, contentment will be sidelined and anger will take over the game.

The more of your players you know about, the more control you have over the game. When you know all your players and are familiar with exactly what they do (and the consequences they create), you can play the best game possible. You have at your command the entire spectrum of your capabilities. However, in the process of getting to know all your players well, you may decide that you do not want to play some of them at all. In fact, you want to retire them from the team. If you find that the consequences some of your players create are always painful for you to experience, you will avoid playing them and begin to choose players that create different consequences. If you find that the consequences other players create are always joyful, you will play those players more and more. Eventually, they will be the only players you send onto the court. No matter what other coaches play, you will choose players that create the consequences that you want to create.

The players that you decide to retire do not leave the team willingly. They are accustomed to playing when they choose. Before you became aware of them, they stepped into the game without your opposition and dominated it at will. After you become aware of them, they forcefully demand to be played. The more you choose other players, the more forceful their demands become. If the player is anger, it becomes enraged. If it is jealousy, its jealousy becomes fierce. It is tempting to play these mutinous players in order not to feel their jealousy, rage, vengefulness, and so on, which are all painful. However, the consequences that they create on the court will always be painful when you encounter them.

Either you encounter the pain of their jealousy, rage, vengefulness, etc., when you do not play them, or you play them and encounter the pain of the consequences that they create for you. After a few seasons as coach, your experience will show you that as painful as it is not to play these players, the pain that they create for you when they play is even greater. You can avoid their pain momentarily (by choosing to play them again and again), but each time you play them, the consequences of playing them bring you more pain. Eventually, you will develop the ability to face these difficult players and tell them the news that they do everything in their power to avoid hearing: "You are not going to play today. You will be on the bench while I play kindness, patience, gratitude, or appreciation" (or any of the players that create consequences for you that are constructive and feel wonderful).

The more you decline to play the players that create destructive and painful consequences, the more they object. They stomp up and down along the sideline shouting, screaming obscenities, belittling you, judging you harshly, weeping, and doing all they can to distract you from the game and to convince or manipulate you into putting them back on the court, but without opportunities to play they begin to get rusty. This doesn't happen quickly, but it happens. They weaken from lack of exercise, and their focus becomes diffuse. They remain forcefully present—usually for a long time—all the while losing strength and skill. They become less intimidating and less distracting. Even when they are still intimidating and painful to experience, their intimidation and painful presence help you develop the ability to be with them, see them, hear them, feel their best efforts to get back into the game, and still choose to play other players.

At this point, you are beginning to master the game, choosing at each moment the best player to send onto the court and accepting responsibility with each choice for the consequences that player creates for you.

The players that create destructive and painful consequences for you, that refuse to be sidelined until you become aware of them and take them out of the game, are the frightened parts of your personality. Every one of them—anger, jealousy, rage, vengefulness, anxiety, fear, feelings of superiority and inferiority, the need to please others or to shout louder, to shop for what they do not need, eat what they do not need, smoke, gamble, watch pornography, drink alcohol, abuse drugs, and on and on—originates in fear. The list of the frightened parts of your personality is as long as the list of your painful emotions and obsessions, compulsions, and addictions. They all have three things in common:

1. They express fear.

2. They are painful to experience.

3. They create painful, destructive consequences.

They are also central to your spiritual development.

The fear-based parts of your personality are the parts that you were born to heal. They are your avenues to spiritual growth (not your obstacles). You cannot develop spiritually and remain vengeful, enraged, jealous, caught in the addictive sexual energy current, unable to stop eating or feeling overwhelmed, and so on. As long as these players are able to decide for themselves (unchallenged by you) when they will enter the game, you cannot grow spiritually. You can meditate, pray, visualize, chant, listen to sermons, be inspired, and read scriptures, but while your anger, jealousy, vengefulness, and fear (for example, your righteousness, judgments, and need for agreement) remain outside of your awareness, much less your control, they will erupt into your life at will, creating destructive and painful consequences for you, and each time you encounter one of those consequences, a frightened part of your personality again steps into the game, creating more painful consequences, and so on. (Buddhists call this process samsara, the Sea of Suffering, or the Wheel of Life.)

Painful experiences endlessly activate frightened parts of your personality, which in turn create more painful experiences until you intervene. Without your intervention, your life unfolds robotically as it has in the past from one painful experience to another. You appear to be at the mercy of chance, praying for good luck and desperately seeking to avoid more pain. These are the experiences of a victim. In other words, unskilled coaches do not realize their central role in the game of "Life." They watch as passive observers, unaware that they are choosing which players will step onto the court and which will not.

Spiritual growth requires locating, experiencing, and challenging (choosing not to play) the frightened parts of your personality. The more you ignore them (repress, suppress, or deny your painful emotions), the more they play, and the more painful consequences you encounter. When I first realized that "spiritual growth" requires me to become aware of everything that I experience, including my painful emotions and feelings of inadequacy, ugliness, unlovability, and shame (players on my team), I felt crushed and defeated (more players). My last hope of transcending my painful experiences, ascending above them, detouring around them, meditating or praying them away, or in some manner avoiding them was shattered. That realization was my first glimpse of myself as a coach, and I did not like the role. I still wanted someone or something to remove the pain and emptiness from my life, and I did not want to look at the possibility (the reality) that I was responsible for that job.

The players that feel good to experience and that create healthy consequences which are pleasing to encounter are the loving parts of your personality. When they are active you become patient, caring, joyful, content, kind, interested in others, and grateful for your life. You have no memory of fear. You know that you are alive for a purpose and that what you are doing serves that purpose. You have everything you need, and you are fully engaged in the present moment.

You cannot play a loving part of your personality and a frightened part at the same time. Playing patience, for example, sidelines impatience. The more you play patience, the stronger it becomes while impatience loses strength. After a while impatience begins to atrophy, the frequency and intensity of its demands diminish, and eventually it loses the ability to impose itself on you. Then it becomes too weak even to influence you. It continues to object to being on the bench, but it can no longer play unless you decide to play it.

As you become aware of yourself as a coach, among the first things you notice are how many frightened parts of your personality are on the team and how often they play. This is always an unexpected and disturbing discovery. If you thought of yourself as gentle and caring, for example, you will be surprised to discover players on your team (parts of your personality) that are enraged and brutal. If you are indignant at the idea of prostitution, for example, you will be surprised to discover (like many clergymen who have campaigned viscerally against prostitution) that one of the players on your team is addicted to sex.

Sometimes an unaware coach gets a glimpse of players on her team that she did not expect to see and refuses to look again because she does not want to confirm what she is not willing to believe. The more she refuses, the more those players step onto the court at their pleasure, and the more painful consequences she encounters. Sooner or later she will make the connection between her painful experiences and her choice of players, even if she does not want to admit that she has players that create painful consequences for her, and begin to schedule let's-get-acquainted meetings with each of her players.

Making this connection usually takes a long time and many encounters with many painful consequences, but it does not have to. If you understand the game of "Life" and your role in it as a coach, you will not need to wait until the accumulated agony of countless painful consequences overwhelms you and you at last begin to explore the relationship between your pain and your choice of players.

Multisensory perception illuminates your role, abilities, and responsibilities as a coach. It does not require you to play this player or that, create this consequence or that, or even become acquainted with your team. Instead it reveals the potential of a life unlike any you have experienced before, with challenges unlike any you have experienced before, and with rewards unlike any you have imagined.

7

Joy vs. Happiness

Opening the shutters, raising the blinds, and pulling back the curtains allows light into a dark room. The light is not created by removing the obstructions. It exists along with the obstructions, and when they are gone, the light remains. Who has not felt the joy of brilliant sunlight flooding darkness, eradicating despair, defining with unmistakable certainty all that it illuminates? This is the journey from grief into acceptance, ignorance into knowledge, doubt into trust, and fear into love. It is the parting of the clouds, the burning away of the mist, and vibrant colors replacing gray. What prevented the warmth, color, knowledge, and certainty is gone, and in its place appears all that was missing. Even the longest nights come to an end, and those who were farthest from the sun in the depth of the night come closest to it the following noon. Obstructions to the sun come and go. The light of the sun is constant.

Striving to create joy is like striving to create sunlight. It is as impossible as it is unnecessary. The journey from darkness to light takes countless forms, but at the heart of each is a transformation that occurs when obstructions to joy are removed. Your obstructions to joy are not things that you think you need and lack such as money, sex, recognition, influence, or anything else. Your obstacles to joy are frightened parts of your personality that need these things in order to feel safe and valuable. They prevent you from experiencing joy the same way that blinds and curtains keep sunlight from a room.

Michelangelo Buonarroti (1475–1564) was one of the greatest figures in the Italian Renaissance and perhaps the greatest sculptor in the history of art. One of his most famous works is the giant statue (seventeen feet high) of David, the young Israelite, as he readies himself to confront Goliath. He is armed only with a sling in one hand and a stone in the other, his face conveys alertness and tension, his young body is strong and athletic. I have seen this amazing sculpture. The skin is so smooth, the musculature so exquisitely defined, the curly hair and worried face so real in appearance that they defy the imagination to reduce them to stone and skill.

Michelangelo saw this magnificent figure within the huge block of marble before his chisel touched the surface, and he passionately labored to remove the stone that held it captive. This was Michelangelo's experience of sculpting. He saw the figure imprisoned in the block, and by removing excess stone he freed it. He completed his first Pietà, perhaps the most famous sculpture in the Western world (and still in its original place in St. Peter's Basilica), in his midtwenties. From then through his late eighties this brilliant, creative, tormented, and angry man liberated from stone some of the most elegant and profoundly human figures in the history of art. Perhaps as he vigorously attacked the blocks that imprisoned them, he sought to destroy the prison that held him captive from his youth and in which he died. As he grew older, his temper did not diminish, nor his disposition soften. Dissatisfied with a work, he turned his rage on one of his last sculptures, the Florentine Pietà (carved for his own tomb), breaking off a leg and an arm from the figure of Christ and one of the Virgin Mary's hands with a hammer. Loneliness, sorrow, and anger remained his companions unto death, as they had been through his life.

Michelangelo lived large the painful stereotype of the artist as isolated, temperamental, and suffering that is only now being replaced with the more accurate perception of the artist as aware, responsible, intuitive, courageous enough to engage Life fully in the present moment, wise enough to see herself and others clearly, and compassionate enough to care for all. What you do not see within you, you see outside of you. You despise in others the greed or lust that you deny in yourself. You blame others for the sorrow that you will not address in yourself and push them further away. The prison that you strive to dismantle in front of your eyes mirrors the real prison behind your eyes that holds you captive. Michelangelo continued to remove the stone that imprisoned beauty in blocks of marble until he died, but he remained until death a prisoner of his anger and harsh judgments. "I . . . have no friends, nor do I want any," he wrote in a letter. His self-criticism, which intensified as he grew old, was ruthless, and he rarely finished his later sculptures.

Within this difficult personality lived also sensitivity and compassion, wisdom and perception of Divinity, and the intelligence of genius—abundant in his poetry and correspondence—yet his life was nearly devoid of sensitive relationships and compassionate actions. He lived alone, becoming even more reclusive in old age, and argued throughout his life with servants, fellow artists (such as Leonardo da Vinci), and popes. The beauty that he saw in marble existed within him as well, but he never sought to reveal, illuminate, or share it as he did the figures that he freed from stone. He did not challenge his anger or his need to object, find fault, and impose himself. He chose isolation instead of companionship, disdain instead of appreciation, and argument instead of communication. In other words, he chose fear instead of love. This choice is not always apparent as a choice, but it is a choice nonetheless.

Impulses that seem irresistible—such as to shout, blame, judge, and seek revenge—are experiences of fear-based parts of your personality. Some of them are so familiar that they feel like "who I am." For example, "I am angry, I have always been angry, and I always will be angry," and "I never interrupt people, I always let them speak first, act first, and decide first." These are the parts of your personality that create destructive and painful consequences that, when you encounter them, reactivate those same parts (and you become angry and shout again; feel invisible and defer again, and so on). You can choose not to shout or defer, as Michelangelo could have chosen not to argue or withdraw, if you are aware of the possibility in the moment.

Multisensory perception enables you to see this possibility—the choice between a frightened part of your personality and a loving part of your personality. Painful physical sensations in certain areas of your body, judgmental thoughts, and the intention to manipulate and control external circumstances all inform you that a frightened part of your personality is active. Choosing a loving part of your personality when you are upset instead of a frightened part frees joy in the same way that Michelangelo's chisels and mallets freed the beauty that he saw in blocks of stone. The frightened parts of your personality (your fears) are the stone. The loving parts of your personality (your joy) are the beauty. They remain in prison until you free them.

Frightened parts of your personality create external power. When you allow a frightened part of your personality to speak or act for you, it creates consequences that are painful to encounter. For example, I pushed colleagues away with disdain, judgment, and jealousy for years, all the while creating a distance between us that was painful and confusing to me. Feeling superior was one of the ways that I masked (from myself) the pain of my fear (terror) of life and people. I found fault with them, judged their deficiencies, and saw myself as better. I was imprisoned by this frightened part of my personality as much as the *David* was imprisoned in marble before Michelangelo freed it.

Sex was another way that I masked the pain of powerlessness. No matter how much I had, I craved more. Even when I was exhausted from sex, I craved more. I imagined myself as a manly, admirable, sexual being, and my sexual encounters and desperate searches for them prevented me from acknowledging, much less experiencing, how ugly, defective, unlovable, and unable to love I felt myself to be. Each sexual encounter temporarily relieved me from these painful experiences, and then the search began again. As before, I was imprisoned by this frightened part of my personality as surely as the *David* was a prisoner in marble, except that no sculptor could free me.

The most that a frightened part of your personality can offer you is temporary relief from the pain of powerlessness. For example, when you long for a new car (dress, house, partner, etc.), you feel wonderful when you get it. Thoughts of inadequacy and unworthiness disappear. You feel more attractive, alive, witty, and sexual. Despair, depression, longing, wanting, and needing vanish. Getting what a frightened part of your personality wants brings out the sun, so to speak, and the fog disappears. This is happiness. You feel good to be relieved of pain, but the relief does not last. If your new car is stolen, your new house has termites, or your new partner does not want to be with you, the sun disappears and the fog returns. When a frightened part of your personality gets what it wants, the pain of powerlessness immediately disappears (happiness). When it does not get what it wants, or loses what it has, the pain immediately returns (happiness disappears).

Happiness depends on what happens outside of you, which is beyond your control, and frightened parts of your personality forever attempt to control it (this is the pursuit of external power). When they succeed, you are happy. When they fail (a relationship dissolves, you lose your job, you are offended by a clerk, etc.), you are unhappy (the pain of powerlessness returns).

The loving parts of your personality are content, grateful, patient, appreciative, caring, and more. They are interested in others. They do not judge others or themselves. They are not confined by fear. The more you experience them, the more you experience joy. When you experience them continually, you experience joy continually. Awe of a sunset, sunrise, the ocean, a mountain, the beauty of another soul, the tenderness of a touch, and the warmth of a smile undistorted by fear are experiences of joy. Joy is knowing why you are alive and being grateful to be living. It is fulfillment in the present moment without end. The Universe sings with joy, and when you free yourself from the frightened parts of your personality you join the song.

Acting with a loving part of your personality when a frightened part of your personality is active (for example, wanting to shout in anger and choosing instead to listen because you do not want to be controlled by your anger) challenges that frightened part. The more you challenge it, the more it loses its control over you. You still become angry, but the more you challenge the frightened part of your personality that is angry, the less intensely you are compelled to act or speak in anger, and the more you are free to act and speak from a loving part of your personality. Eventually the control over you by the frightened part of your personality that is angry disappears altogether.

Challenging a frightened part of your personality requires experiencing the pain of powerlessness and, at the same time, choosing differently than it habitually chooses (for example, not shouting, disdaining, or withdrawing emotionally). Each time you challenge a frightened part of your personality, you remove chips from the walls of your prison. Michelangelo did not create his magnificent sculptures with a few blows. He created them one hammer strike at a time, day after day and often night after night, chipping pieces of marble away with each blow. You free your joy in the same way. Your intention is your chisel, and your will is your mallet. Each choice to act with a frightened part of your personality leaves the walls of your prison untouched and intact. Each choice to act with a loving part of your personality sends pieces of marble flying, thinning the walls and revealing the joy within you.

The more you diminish the power of the frightened parts of your personality over you, the more joy you experience. No one can do this for you, and you cannot do it for others. When you choose to control or manipulate others (pursue external power), you reinforce the marble that encases your joy. When you choose to change yourself (create authentic power), you free it. The more you free your joy, the more it becomes part of your experience. Eventually, only joy remains.

Joy is permanent. Happiness is temporary. Joy depends upon what happens inside of you. Happiness depends upon what happens outside of you. Bringing joy into your life requires you to become an artist and your life to become your art.

You cannot create joy, but you do not need to. The path is simpler. You need only remove obstructions to it. When the shutters, blinds, and curtains of your life (the frightened parts of your personality) are opened slightly and you peek out (experiment with creating authentic power), joy makes its way into your life. When you open them wide (challenge the frightened parts of your personality until their control over you disintegrates), joy floods into your life like sunlight. Joy versus happiness is a choice. It occurs many times each day, each hour, and sometimes each minute. Only you can choose to challenge and heal a frightened part of your personality (respond) when you are angry, jealous, vengeful, anxious, etc., or to strengthen it (react). Only you can choose to cultivate and develop a loving part of your personality when you are patient, grateful, caring, appreciative, etc. (act on it), or to weaken it (ignore it).

Happiness requires changing circumstances, including people. Joy requires changing yourself.

8

Authentic Power

The more you cultivate loving parts of your personality and challenge frightened parts, the more your personality becomes aligned with your soul. Eventually, the frightened parts of your personality lose their control over you and the loving parts create without limitation. Fear disappears. Your experiences become meaningful. Your attention is in the never-ending miracle of the eternal present moment. Your relationships transform. You are not "connected" to others any more than you are "connected" to your arm, hand, or heart. You are part of them, and they are part of you. When they hurt, you feel them. When they are healthy, you are healthy.

Humbleness, clarity, forgiveness, and love replace fear. The world becomes a friendly place. You see the struggles and spiritual potential of others and the complexity and richness of their lives, even if they are not aware of them. Superiority gives way to appreciation. Inferiority disappears. The energy of your soul flows effortlessly through you into the Earth school like the breath of a musician through a flute. Neither you nor others can tell where your personality ends and your soul begins. Gratitude, joy, meaning, and bliss fill your days. The seasons of your life come and go, carrying you forward like a river returning to the sea.

You consult intuition, choose your intentions consciously, move forward with an empowered heart, and act without attachment to the outcome. You do not presume to know how the Universe works or question the wisdom and compassion that shape your experiences according to the choices that you have made. You do your part and trust your nonphysical guides and Teachers to do theirs, take responsibility for your choices, and strive to contribute compassionately and wisely to Life. Each moment is full and complete. You think in terms of causes (intentions) and effects (experiences) instead of right and wrong, good and bad, fortunate and unfortunate. You know that a factor of karma is involved in your experiences, and so you do not take them personally. You give without expectation and receive without reservation. All that you need is given to you. This is authentic power.

Many people have brief and spontaneous experiences of authentic power, for example, while cooking a meal, nursing a child, painting a canvas, or caring for a parent. Experiences of authentic power are the most fulfilling that your life can offer you. They are the nectar of the human experience. You live in the perfection of the Universe, fully engaged and aware. These experiences can be created consciously, and creating them is our new evolutionary requirement.

As the soul becomes visible in the awareness of millions of individuals, a new center of gravity is developing in the human experience. The creation of authentic power is replacing the pursuit of external power. Aligning personality with soul—with harmony, cooperation, sharing, and reverence for Life—is becoming the new polestar by which we navigate through our lives. Without this new star, uncharted reefs, wild seas, typhoons, and unwanted calms delay and divert us from our common goal—a life of clarity, humbleness, forgiveness, and love. Winds of anger, jealousy, and vengefulness shred sails, break masts, and tear ships apart. Apathy, lethargy, and despair leave them adrift. Superiority and inferiority, entitlement and the need to please pull compasses and ships alike off course.

The great transformation in consciousness that is reshaping human experience reveals a larger fabric of Life (nonphysical reality), offers a new potential (authentic power), and illuminates a new evolutionary requirement (spiritual growth). None can take its measure. Nothing except the genesis of humanity can compare with it. A five-sensory humanity in pursuit of external power (surviving by manipulating and controlling circumstances) is becoming a multisensory humanity in pursuit of authentic power (evolving by aligning personality with soul).

As magnificent as this transformation is, it will not make you patient, caring, or loving. If anger disrupts your life before you become multisensory, it will continue to disrupt your life when you become multisensory. If you exploit others before you become multisensory, you will continue to exploit them when you become multisensory. If you are tormented by jealousy, multisensory perception will not ease your torment. Multisensory perception allows you to see more and experience more, but it cannot transform you from an unempowered personality into an empowered personality. That is your responsibility.

For the first time human evolution requires conscious choice—specifically, your conscious choice. Only you can choose to experience the pain of powerlessness in your body when you are upset (for example, feeling overwhelmed, inadequate, guilty, or resentful) and challenge a frightened part of your personality (respond) instead of react. Only you can make different and healthy choices instead of overeating, smoking, watching pornography, shopping, gambling, drinking alcohol, using drugs, or having mindless sex. Only you can choose to use your emotions, including the most painful, to grow spiritually instead of masking them with obsessive thoughts, compulsive actions, and addictive behaviors.

Multisensory humans are as challenged by spiritual growth as five-sensory humans were challenged by survival, but in different ways. Surviving does not require conscious choices. At night on patrol in the Laotian jungle I did not need to choose to survive. I clung to my training and mission like a man in an angry sea to a life rope, all thoughts, all choices, all awareness focused by the closeness of death. Challenging and healing frightened parts of your personality requires conscious choices, and you cannot grow spiritually without challenging and healing them.

Multisensory perception moves choice (your choice) to stage center in your evolution and the evolution of humanity. Choice of intention becomes your instrument, you become the musician, and your life becomes the music. If the notes you hear are cold, hard, and discordant, you can change the composition without stopping the music. You can never stop the music, but you can choose the music. If the notes inspire you and reveal beautiful vistas, you can play more.

When you travel in the direction that your soul wants to go, you fill with meaning. When you travel in other directions, meaning drains from your life. When you travel in the opposite direction, your life empties of meaning. Your soul wants harmony, cooperation, sharing, and reverence for Life. It wants you to create them in your life—to become a beacon to fellow students in the Earth school and allow them to become beacons to you. Giving the gifts that you were born to give (traveling in the direction that your soul wants to travel) brings you more gifts to give. The creativity of the Universe is inexhaustible, and therefore, so is yours.

Healing frightened parts of your personality and cultivating loving parts of your personality transform the collective consciousness with the power of your own. Instead of imploding under the fear of the collective, you change the consciousness of the collective with your own consciousness. Every great soul has walked this path. Now our evolution requires each of us to choose it. What is in us is in the whole, and therefore, each of us is ultimately responsible for the whole. The changes that you create in yourself are the changes that you create in the world. Choosing cooperation instead of competition, sharing instead of hoarding, harmony instead of discord, and reverence for Life instead of exploitation changes you, and it changes the whole at the same time.

When you ask yourself, "What difference can I make? Why should I be kind when others are cruel? How can my choices change the world?" you disempower yourself. From the multisensory perspective, these questions become "How can my choices not change the world?" You disempower yourself by waiting for a "critical mass" to transform the world. You will not change while you wait—the frightened parts of your personality will remain unchallenged—and the fear in the collective consciousness will remain unchallenged also. Your choices, one by one, to create authentic power instead of pursue external power affect the health of the whole just as the health of one part of a body affects all of its parts.

No individual in the Earth school is separate from the activities in it, even the most repulsive. The hatred that led young Saudi Arabian men to fly planes full of people into the World Trade Center and the Pentagon was fueled by our hatred. Their righteousness and disregard for Life was fueled by our righteousness and disregard for others. Those who exploit the Earth and life on it are fueled by our intentions to gain the most for the least—from a circumstance, employee, job, friend, partner, or neighbor.

When you create authentic power you determine what is healthy for you and what is not; what is worthy of your interest and what is not. You decide which of your sensations, thoughts, and intentions originate in love and which originate in fear. You become the authority in your life, and your life becomes a continual meditation. Every experience offers you an opportunity to create authentic power or pursue external power.

The journey to authentic power is the journey that you were born to take. Only you can decide when to begin it, and only you can do the work to complete it, but it is not a journey that you can take alone.

9

Soul Summary

I have put an Executive Summary for the Soul at the end of each section and wherever one seems useful. These Soul Summaries recap what has come before, sometimes give a perspective that is not in the chapter(s), and sometimes lead into what is coming next. I hope you find them helpful. They are designed to make the concepts and examples more usable and relevant. One of my spiritual partners is a senior executive at a large electronics firm. He tells his engineers when they excitedly present a new concept or product to him, "Explain to me so my mom would understand." I hope these Soul Summaries will help you explain what you are learning to Mom (or your spouse, children, friends, and coworkers).

SPIRITUAL PARTNERSHIPS—WHY

- Human consciousness has changed.
- We can experience more than the five senses detect.
- This is multisensory perception.
- Everyone will be multisensory in a few generations.
- This is a big change—it has not happened to the entire human species before.
- We can sense ourselves as personalities and souls at the same time.
- We can know things we couldn't before—meaning, information, reasons for past events, etc.
- Everyone feels unworthy and defective. This is very painful.

- Intentions are very important (they create consequences).
- We are responsible for what we create.
- Happiness depends on what happens outside of us.
- Joy depends on what happens inside of us.
- Parts of our personalities make us feel unworthy and defective.
- We can change those parts (instead of other people).
- This is creating authentic power.
- We are each responsible for creating authentic power.

The ground rules of a life on the Earth have changed, and these changes are permanent. Old ways of doing things don't work anymore, or they work but produce experiences we don't want. Old ways of relating don't work anymore, either. The new consciousness brings a new type of relationship that is as different from the old type as the new, multisensory consciousness is from the old, five-sensory consciousness. This new type of relationship is coming up next (in this book and in your life).

WHAT

10

The End of Friendship

A mature friendship is the ultimate accomplishment of
five-sensory humans. It is distinct from every other
five-sensory form of relationship, including marriages
and family relationships. Mature friendships emerge from a
developmental process that cannot be short-circuited. In other
words, they require work, mutual care, and commitment. Casual
friendships are common and transitory. They are experiences of
mutual attraction based upon limited perceptions and limited
knowledge of a new friend, or friends. For example, women meet
at a function for parents, men meet at a sports event, or students
meet in a class, and an attraction arises that makes all involved
feel better and safe. There are always commonalities that create
this experience of safety, for example, a shared religion, spiritual
practice, interest in athletics, or challenges of parenting. Often
there are larger commonalities, such as race, nationality, sex,
culture, and economic circumstance. It is much less common for
a wealthy white businessperson to create a casual friendship with
a brown immigrant farmworker than with another wealthy white
businessperson, and vice versa.

Casual friendships are not durable. They come and go, often
quickly, and are replaced by other equally superficial relationships. The discovery that a casual friend is gay or lesbian, Republican or Democrat, Muslim or Jew, poor or rich is often enough to
end the relationship. The more that casual friends learn about one
another, the more different they appear to one another than their
initial, uninformed perceptions presented. New awarenesses
make one or more of the casual friends uncomfortable, and a dis-

tance appears between them. The urge to continue the relationship lessens and then disappears. An impulse toward intimacy and openness is replaced by a more formal and less meaningful interaction. A casual friendship is one step above generally friendly behavior. It is the mutual appreciation of friendly behavior fortified by the appearance of common experiences that makes a possible relationship appear safe and supportive.

Casual friendships are analogous to interactions between children. They easily become upset with one another over whose toy belongs to whom or who got more candy. They run and play together until a misunderstanding triggers anger, disappointment, or fear. Then their behavior changes quickly and often dramatically. This happens among adults when they discover differences between them that they did not expect or want, for example, that one of them becomes loud and insensitive—or sullen and withdrawn—when drinking, and drinks frequently; or smokes and smells of tobacco; or is (or is not) a vegetarian; and so on. The casual friendship returns to friendly behavior at best or transforms into judgment and hostility at worst. Every life is filled with transient casual friendships, each an attraction to the potential security of sameness; a tentative exploration of sameness; an attempt to find refuge in sameness.

A friendship begins to mature when unexpected differences and new perceptions arise and the desire to keep the connection is greater than the desire to end it. This happens when one or more of the newly revealed individuals (the gay, lesbian, Republican, Democrat, etc.) reaches out in a meaningful way and touches a deeper current in the other or others. For example, she comes to the hospital to visit your dying mother, or offers to shop for groceries for you while you are with your mother, or brings you the toy that you wanted for your child and couldn't find. This is the magic movement, the new element that transforms a casual friendship into a friendship. One individual cares enough about another to proactively support the other, and if the other is receptive, that support opens a doorway. You enter one another's lives, even if briefly. The choice to support the well-being of another creates a potential that did not previously exist.

The proffered and received support may appear small, such as a birthday card or the offer of a ride home that takes the driver out of her way, but the intention behind it is large. The intention distinguishes love from fear and injects the former into the relationship, even if the friends do not think in terms of loving one another. Meetings between friends of this type cease to be entirely spontaneous—such as chance meetings at the coffee shop, or at work—and become planned and anticipated. You call and are called. You begin to share about yourselves in ways that are comfortable for you both, and you begin to know about one another.

Our granddaughter plays on a volleyball team that practices daily. Linda and I go to her games when we visit, and we have met the parents of some of her teammates that way. Our interactions are mostly examples of friendly behavior, but some are developing into casual friendships—we enjoy encountering some of the parents at the games, and they enjoy seeing us. Each casual friendship holds the potential for maturing into a more durable friendship. It requires only that one of the casual friends make the needs of another, at least temporarily, as important as her own.

The more that casual friends are together, the more they learn about each other. For example, they see in each other anger, jealousy, or the need to gossip as well as tenderness and sensitivity, or the lack of them, yet their care for each other allows them to accept these behaviors, even though they previously would have rejected them. They see the struggles and achievements, moments of vulnerability and moments of defensiveness, and times of openness and joy in each other. As their care for each other grows they learn more about each other's fears and aspirations and values and prejudices. Their differences and similarities become clear. They experience challenges and joy with each other. Eventually they come to accept each other and, in some cases, cherish each other. They are there for each other. Neither time nor distance can diminish their closeness. Each resides in the other's heart.

This is as close to "friends for life" as five-sensory individuals can come, yet these friendships have limits. A sudden descent into alcoholism, drug abuse, emotional instability, or violence can create a chasm between friends. Even mature friendships fade when values change and diverge. When one friend, for example, remains single and a sexual predator and the other marries and devotes himself to his family, a connection remains between them, but the vibrant experiences of a mature friendship are replaced by sentimental attachment to a relationship that no longer exists.

Friendship is an old-type relationship that was designed for, and served the evolution of, five-sensory humans. It allows bonding, deep connections, mutual appreciation, and emotional closeness among individuals who are evolving through the pursuit of external power. It is the natural expression of love, tailored for individuals who are limited in their perception to the five senses. Like all old-type relationships, it enhances the pursuit of external power. It belongs to the category of interaction that originates in the need to join with others in order to accomplish a goal that none alone can achieve.

Friends look to one another to help them avoid the pain of powerlessness. They support one another in their sorrow and celebrate their accomplishments without examining the interior causes of their sorrow and happiness. They see only physical causes and physical effects. They seek surcease of suffering in the alteration of physical circumstances—for example, helping a friend reestablish a relationship or find another job—without exploring the parts of his personality that generate pain and destructive consequences. They assist one another in justifying distress, for example, "I don't blame you for being angry; I would be angry, too," and "What a cruel thing, after all that you did for her." They validate the experiences of frightened parts of the personality, "Of course you feel upset; anyone would," and "It is natural to be afraid (be lonely, want revenge, etc.)." They empathize and sympathize, for example, "I lost my mother, too," "How terrible; she just walked out!" and "How could he betray you like that!"

The ways that five-sensory individuals attempt to uplift one another are as numerous as the experiences of frightened parts of the personality. They give advice ("When my wife left, I . . ."); attempt to solve one another's problems ("You should see my doctor . . ."); and caretake ("Everything will be all right, wait and see . . ."). Friends think in terms of failure and success instead of cause and effect, choice and responsibility. When one fails, others cheer her up without helping her learn about herself from her experience. When she succeeds, they celebrate with her without helping her learn about herself from her experience. They are often unaware of intentions—their own or others'—and therefore they are not able to relate choices of intention to consequences. Good fortune (friends celebrate this) and bad luck (friends lament this) visit each without apparent cause—random blessings and curses with no visible connection to the blessed or cursed friend. These are the shared contents of a friendship.

Friends are limited to the perspective of the personal. In other words, they take their interactions personally. They are offended or comforted by the actions of one another without exploring the origins of their offense or comfort apart from physical circumstances and without considering the factor of karma. They approve (judge) or disapprove (judge) one another. Frightened parts of one personality interact with frightened parts of others, creating an experience of safety that is anchored in their common thoughts, beliefs, and actions. For example, Christians feel more comfortable with one another than with non-Christians, white people feel more comfortable with one another than with people of other colors, athletes feel more comfortable with one another than with intellectuals, and so on.

Friends support one another, but their support is different from the support that multisensory humans require. Friends see support as assistance in achieving their goals, consolation when they are grieving, sympathy when they are in pain, empathy when they are upset, and shared pleasure when they are happy. They expect certain behaviors from one another and react when their expectations are not met. They do not understand, or see, that their reactions, such as tears, anger, jealousy, and emotional withdrawal, are attempts to manipulate one another and so the interior causes of their reactions (frightened parts of the personality) remain unchallenged. Friends assume that the causes of emotional distress are external, and they strive (are mutually manipulated) to avoid triggering reactions in one another. In other words, they learn to maneuver around the frightened parts of one another's personalities, for example, by not saying things that might trigger anger, sorrow, withdrawal, or jealousy. They become comfortable with one another and are careful not to rock the boat in a way that will jeopardize the mutual comfort that they value.

When friends work through disagreements with apologies, explanations, sympathy, and empathy, they become closer and their shared experience of safety and comfort deepens. However, the frightened parts of their personalities are not recognized or healed, and future reactions are insured. Each reaction is experienced as a threat to the friendship (which it is) rather than an opportunity to find and heal the interior cause of it.

Now that we are becoming multisensory, the limitations of friendship are becoming visible. The goal of five-sensory humans (survival) is not the goal of multisensory humans (spiritual growth). The means of achieving the goal of five-sensory humans (external power) is not the means of achieving the goal of multisensory humans (authentic power). Everything in the human experience is changing as we transit from a five-sensory humanity into a multisensory humanity, including our relationships. In the process, friendship is being replaced with a new, more spiritually accurate relationship that is designed for, and serves the evolution of, multisensory humans.

When I lived in a small mountain community I belonged to a men's group that met weekly for two years. There were only four of us in the group, and we became very close. We came to cherish one another and our time together. We mountain biked, skied, hiked, and explored the wilderness together. We shared our homes with each other, dined together, and called upon one another for help, such as when I returned from a trip and found my water pipes frozen. We argued and reconciled, sympathized, empathized, cajoled, and consoled one another. In short, we shared our lives and enriched one another immensely.

Our group broke up when one of the men moved away, but my friendship with him remained strong and close. I felt that I knew him and he knew me. That is why I was shocked into numbness when I heard that he had hanged himself. I couldn't answer the voice on the phone (a member of our group) or put the phone down. I wanted to throw up, and at the same time I knew it was because I could not digest what I had heard. The next hours were tumultuous. First came tears and then fierce anger. "Why did you do this? Do you think you are the only one in the world? Do you think that others don't have feelings? What about us? What about me? You didn't even say good-bye." Then came a tidal wave of grief. I cried without being willing or able to stop.

The evening before, Linda and I had attended a performance of monks from a Tibetan monastery in India and been touched by the power of their chanting. Now, after hearing of my friend's death, even though it was late, I wanted to visit them! We called their hosts, and they invited us to their home. When we arrived the monks were very much awake and lively. I did my best to explain the suicide of my friend to the abbot and why we were there (although I did not know). Talking was difficult because each new wave of grief choked me, and all I could do was halt for the moment and try to regain my breath and voice. When I finished, the abbot, who had been listening closely, said simply, "Since you cannot do anything more for your friend, why not relax? Will you join us for dinner?" I could not have anticipated the effect of his words on me. For a moment, my grief lifted. His invitation felt very appropriate and his observation evident. Although a part of me (a frightened part) again wanted to grieve, I decided to stay for dinner and Linda agreed.

That decision was an important one for me. The monks carried a picture of my friend (my best picture of him) back to India to put in their temple for a year, and I still remember the unexpected late-night meal that Linda and I shared with twenty laughing, lighthearted companions on the day that one of my dearest friends took his life. I do not know if the monks thought in terms of challenging frightened parts of the personality, but they helped me challenge a frightened part of mine. I still had more tears to cry and sorrow to feel (more experiences of frightened parts of my personality), but I had learned a lesson. I saw that my grief did not depress the monks; instead, their joy elevated me. More than that, I saw that my life did not need to go down a path of pain and sorrow for years. I could choose another path, and, in fact, I did in that moment.

The cheerful monks were much more to me than friends, even though we had not met before. They offered me something different and refreshing and more healing than friendship. They did not console me ("A tragedy like this must be difficult to bear") or sympathize with me ("My brother died this year also") or advise me ("It is better to look ahead than back") or in any way support the fear that was coursing through me, crippling me, paralyzing me, engulfing me. Instead, they showed me a way of being with one another that is far more rewarding, joyful, and empowering than friendship. I had known of this way, and even written about it. They helped me experience it as I had not experienced it before.

This way has a name.

11

Spiritual Partnership

Spiritual partnership is partnership between equals for the purpose of spiritual growth. It is dramatically different from all previous forms of relationship and serves a different purpose. The partners are together in order to help one another grow spiritually instead of enhance their physical comfort and safety. Spiritual partnerships are vehicles that multisensory individuals use to create authentic power and support one another in creating authentic power. They are fundamental parts of our new evolutionary process.

Spiritual partners are interested in one another more than their common objectives. The goal they share is spiritual growth, and each knows that he or she must reach it himself or herself. Their commitment is a promise to their own spiritual development, a determination to move into the fullness of their own potential, to give the gifts that they were born to give. Spiritual partners journey into their deepest fears—their experiences of powerlessness—with the intention to heal them completely. They are the heroes of mythology finding and slaying the dragon, recovering the treasure, and restoring prosperity to the land.

Your dragons live within you, emerging from their lairs as they choose. For example, someone offends you and you become angry. A dragon is out and in the open. Or you withdraw emotionally and judge her silently. Another dragon is out. Or you cannot stop thinking judgmental thoughts or having violent or sexual fantasies, or cannot resist alcohol, food, sex, pornography, or shopping. The dragons are many, and some are quite powerful. All of them are terrifying enough to cause you to flee them at once (by becoming angry, finding fault, drinking alcohol, having sex, shopping, smoking, and so on). No one can slay your dragons for you. You are the hero you have been waiting for. Until you accept this role you will continue to wait, and the longer you wait, the more your dragons will rampage through your life, creating havoc and pain when they choose.

The dragon is not your obsessive judgment, compulsive activity, or addictive behavior. These show you that a dragon is active and making your choices for you. They are indicators, signals to you, that a dragon is at large. To slay your dragon(s) you must journey into its lair (inside you) and challenge it face-to-face. That is why you cannot heal an addiction by wearing nicotine patches or stop overeating by changing your diet. You have not gone into the dragon's lair and challenged it. You have challenged only its activities. The dragon remains. For example, a smoker gives up cigarettes and begins to overeat, or an overeater gives up food and begins to smoke, drink, gamble, or becomes promiscuous. We say that such a person has an "addictive personality," but that is not the case. The dragon has taken a different appearance. Like trying to pick up a drop of mercury with your fingers, you cannot grasp it by changing your behaviors. First the dragon appears one way (such as alcoholism) and then another (such as gambling).

In mythology the dragon comes and goes as it chooses, destroying all that is beautiful and killing every warrior it meets until a hero appears who is willing to risk his life for the king and kingdom. Only he can kill the dragon, if anyone can, and he must do it alone. That is the hero's journey, and only those with courage and commitment can take it. The journey is always long, difficult, and frightening. The hero encounters challenges never experienced before and must call upon his strength, clarity, and determination again and again until at last the dragon is dead. Then he returns triumphant and the land becomes peaceful and prosperous.

Your dragons are the frightened parts of your personality, and you alone can experience and heal them. When the cause of your agony is inside, you must go inside to find and change it. Whether you are young or elderly, male or female, religious or not religious, the journey to your full potential will be long, difficult, and frightening, and only you can make it. Five-sensory friends look for causes of their suffering outside of themselves—in their failed relationships, illnesses, betrayals, and bad luck. They change friends and circumstances but they do not change themselves, and so their interactions with new circumstances and friends produce the same painful experiences. This is the horizontal path. Their dragons remain. Spiritual partners take the vertical path. They change themselves. They slay their own dragons. They do not wait for the impossible, for others to slay their dragons for them.

Individuals in pursuit of authentic power are as courageous as the mightiest warriors, but their goals are different. Their purpose is to recognize the armor they wear (such as irritability, righteousness, superiority, and inferiority) and remove it; to find the weapons they hold (such as anger, jealousy, and vengefulness) and put them down. This is the spiritual path. These individuals naturally form relationships with others who share their purpose, and the relationships that they create are spiritual partnerships. Spiritual partners do not seek allies to change circumstances (external power), but fellow travelers on the journey toward wholeness (authentic power). Courage, integrity, and commitment to their own spiritual growth attract them to one another and keep them together. They trust one another enough to explore their fear and love together. They are brave enough to probe the depths of intimacy.

Multisensory perception gives spiritual partners an impersonal perspective of themselves and their interactions. They no longer see their relationships as means of masking pain but as vehicles to explore and heal the causes of it. The limitations of friendship confine them. They want more than company and security. They want to grow spiritually, to heal the frightened parts of their personalities and cultivate the loving parts. They are not content with controlling their anger in order to keep their relationships together, much less allowing it to devastate their relationships and aspirations. They intend to locate and remove the source of it within themselves. For example, when friends have a painful disagreement, each believes that the other causes her pain and that if only she can get away from the other, she will be happy again. Spiritual partners know that others do not "create my pain" but trigger sources of it within themselves (frightened parts of their personalities) that existed prior to their disagreement and, in fact, prior to their partnership. Instead of blaming one another for painful experiences, such as anger, sadness, and feelings of inadequacy, spiritual partners see one another as colleagues in spiritual growth who activate frightened and loving parts of one another's personalities so that each can heal the frightened parts of his or her own personality and cultivate the loving parts.

The bond between spiritual partners is as real as the bond between mature friends, but for significantly different reasons. Friends seek support from one another when they are buffeted by the winds. Spiritual partners want to know where the winds come from. Friends want to contain the fire. Spiritual partners intend to put it out. Friends bond to ease the journey. Spiritual partners bond to grow spiritually. Friends fear painful interactions. Spiritual partners take responsibility for their experiences and use them to learn about themselves. Friends don't rock the boat. Spiritual partners love to swim. Friends construct comfort zones. Spiritual partners align their personalities with their souls.

For example, when Linda and I first became spiritual partners some of our power struggles lasted for weeks. We created emotional distance from each other. I was shocked at her stubbornness; she resisted my micromanagement. Her rigidity angered me; and my insistence angered her. I fought to control her and she fought to control me in difficult and unwinnable contests. My most painful experiences came not from losing power struggles, but from winning them. The forced submission, buried resentment, and growing distance between us made hollow my every success. Each victory was a defeat. I did not stop to think that my perceptions of Linda might be filtered through my fears (which they always were), or that she might have different intentions than I assumed (which she sometimes did). My goal was to win, and so was hers. Like two gladiators, each armed with weapons of choice, the frightened parts of our personalities engaged each other.

She, armed with withdrawal or tears or a steely smile that pierced my heart, parried my every use of anger, blame, and judgment. Back and forth we sparred, hurting one another, becoming more frightened with each clash. Sometimes we exchanged weapons, and she attacked with anger and I countered with withdrawal. We still get into power struggles, but they last minutes now instead of weeks.

Each time I see how quickly Linda is able to challenge the frightened parts of her personality that bristled with defiance, brooded, or deprecated herself and instead relate to me with loving parts of her personality that are patient, caring, and wise, I am in awe. I know the courage that she plumbs to challenge those parts of her personality (by responding instead of continuing to react), because I know the strength and tenacity of the frightened parts of my personality. Each time she ends a power struggle with her commitment and responsible choice (even if a frightened part of my personality wants to continue it), she models a conscious, determined, deliberate return to love, and each time I find and choose love again after a journey into anger and disdain, I model the same. These are momentous accomplishments. They are journeys that spiritual partners help one another take.

Spiritual partners frequently activate frightened parts of one another's personalities. This is appropriate. Spiritual partnerships are designed to provide the partners opportunities to experience, challenge, and heal frightened parts of their personalities and experience and cultivate loving parts of their personalities in the supportive environment of others who are doing the same. The question is not whether frightened parts of your personality will become active in your spiritual partnerships, but whether or not you will learn from them when they do—experience their painful sensations, observe their judgmental thoughts, see their intentions to manipulate and control, and respond instead of react.

Every individual you encounter has the capability to activate a frightened part of your personality, and many do. When a spiritual partner activates a frightened part of your personality, or you activate one of his or hers, you are both committed to growing spiritually instead of manipulating and controlling one another and this provides all involved an optimal learning experience. The more you use these experiences to create authentic power, the less the frightened parts of your personality control you and the more authentically powerful you become.

Spiritual partners support one another with their courage and commitment to create authentic power, not with knowledge, belief, or teachings. They do not quote authorities, recite passages, or make one another wrong (unless frightened parts of their personalities are active). They are drawn forward by their intention to grow spiritually, not pushed from behind by their fears, such as fear of losing one another and fear of not meeting expectations. They do not persuade, convert, entice, seduce, or convince (these are pursuits of external power), because these endeavors are counterproductive. You cannot heal the fear of another and no one can heal yours, but you can inspire others with your emotional awareness, responsible choices, intuition, and trust in the Universe, and anyone can do the same for you. Spiritual partners do this for one another. They are together because of their choices, not their weaknesses. They intend to change themselves, not one another. They distinguish love from need, care from compulsion, fulfillment from success, joy from happiness, and strive to make healthy choices.

All the frightened parts of their personalities surface in their partnerships, sometimes in concert, because they hold the intention to heal them. These are the same parts of the personality that individuals in old-type relationships try to suppress, repress, deny, or ignore—the parts that are disruptive in their intentions and destructive in their actions. Spiritual partners know that these parts of their personalities illuminate for each what he or she must change in himself or herself in order to move into wholeness. Spiritual partners welcome all of the parts of their personalities, even when they are painful (which the fear-based parts always are). They have no illusions that they can grow spiritually while frightened parts of their personalities are in charge of their lives.

Spiritual partners help one another leap the chasm, again and again, between wanting and doing, wishing and intending, longing and action. The rubber meets the spiritual road when you are furious, want to withdraw emotionally, cannot get out of the bed in the morning, or stop eating, thinking critical thoughts, shopping, or watching pornography and you face what you are feeling (experience the painful sensations in your energy centers) and challenge it instead of indulging it. When you stop before you act habitually (compulsively or addictively) and experience what you are feeling, you enter the dragon's lair. When you respond instead of react, you engage the dragon directly, and the more often you do, the more its power over you diminishes until it disappears.

Just as a child who is terrified of the dark becomes calm when the light is turned on and she can see for herself what is in the room and what is not, fear of your fear disappears when you illuminate and challenge it again and again. You face the monster directly, walk around it, size it up, and see exactly what it is. It still hurts—you are examining the pain of powerlessness up close—but it cannot hurt you more than the destructive consequences that it will create if you allow it to choose your actions and words. When you look directly into its eyes (experience it fully) and choose differently than it would choose, you change yourself and your future. When you choose an intention of your soul, you create authentic power.

Friends, colleagues, classmates, and coworkers avoid the chasm. They are comfortable on the wanting-wishing-longing side of it, and they want you for company. Spiritual partners are drawn to the chasm. Every seeker of truth is. On one side of the chasm lies fear; on the other side lives love; and you make the leap or not with each decision. When you are unaware of your choices, you remain in fear. When you are aware of your fear, you are able to choose differently. You are able to inject consciousness into an otherwise unconscious process and change it. Your spiritual partners help you do that, and you help them.

The more frequently you make the leap, the more practiced you become at it, and the less you fear it. The choice of love instead of fear becomes a continual part of your experience, and eventually, only love remains. Your fear disappears, the chasm disappears, and no leap is required because you are already standing where you need to be, and where you were born to be.

12

Equality

My father owned a jewelry store in a small town in Kansas. Somewhere in his career he acquired an antique diamond scale. My mother kept it on a shelf of our family-room bookcase. I hardly noticed it until after he passed on. When I did, I was impressed by its quality and elegance. The scale itself was enclosed in a handmade glass and mahogany case. The front panel slid up to allow access to the elegant instrument. Its simplicity and beauty made it a work of art for me. Two brass trays, each suspended from an arm poised on a brass column with a fulcrum at the top, balanced one another perfectly. A long, needle-thin pointer, attached to the beam from which the trays hung, descended straight down the full length of the column to the base where vertical markings on a small brass plate showed its slightest deviation from center.

Below the enclosure was a miniature wooden drawer, made with the same care. The drawer contained a small block of wood with small holes of different sizes drilled into it. In each hole a miniature metal weight, molded into the form of a tiny cylinder with a pharmacy-style knob at the top, fit perfectly. A delicate pair of tweezers lay beside the block, and were used to place a diamond onto one of the trays and weights onto the other, one at a time, until the needle again pointed directly downward to center. If too many weights were added to bring the trays into balance again, or too few, the discrepancy was immediately evident.

When both trays were empty, they were level with one another. When a diamond was placed in one tray and its precise weight was placed in the other, they became level again. Only then, at the point of perfect balance, did the long needle point vertically and precisely downward. When either tray was above or below the other, the imbalance was obvious. Perhaps a digital scale could weigh the diamond more precisely, but it would require calibration to insure accuracy. My father's scale does not have this problem. The trays are in perfect balance, full or empty, or they are not. If they are, balance is evident. If they are not, so is the imbalance.

Equality is like that. It exists or it doesn't. In order to see if you feel equal with another person, picture yourself on one tray of an imaginary diamond scale that is large enough to hold people, and picture another person on the other tray. If the trays are level, you are equal. If they are not, you are unequal. Your weight and the weight of the other person do not affect the positions of the trays as they would on a real scale. For example, you may discover that when you put a child on the other tray, your tray, surprisingly, goes up as though the child weighs more than you, or that when you put someone who is heavier than you on the other tray, your tray goes down as though you weigh more.

That is because when you feel superior your tray is always higher than the other tray (you look down on that person). When you feel inferior your tray is always lower (you look up to that person). For example, people who feel superior to their children, or to children in general, always find that their tray is higher when a child is placed on the other tray. These people feel more worthy, important, and valuable than the child (even if they feel that they love the child). People who feel superior in general (or entitled) live on a tray that is always higher regardless of who is on the other tray (for example, a parent or a colleague). On the other hand, people who feel inferior (for instance, need to please) find themselves on the lower tray no matter who is on the other tray (even an abusive partner or insensitive employer). They look up to everyone.

The slightest experience of superiority or inferiority upsets the balance, and one tray sinks below or rises above the other.

The scale always shows your balance (equality) or imbalance (inequality). It is your personal scale. It does not show you the experiences of others. They have their own scales. What they see on their scales is for them. What you see on your scale is for you.

I often discover that my scale is out of balance, no matter how shocked I am at each discovery. The more I explore the frightened parts of my personality, the more I see how superior some of them feel toward women, people who are older, people who are younger, and people who believe, speak, or appear differently than I do. Some of the frightened parts of my personality feel that they have no equal in creation, an extraordinarily arrogant (frightened) and inaccurate perception, but not to them. It is a jolt to me to find that they are prejudiced in ways that I abhor, but they exist and until I became aware of them, I could not challenge them and they determined my actions.

As you become aware of the different parts of your personality, you may discover that your scale is out of balance as frequently as I discovered mine to be, but perhaps in different ways. For example, you may discover a frightened part of your personality that also feels it has no equal in creation, but in the opposite way—it feels inferior to all of creation. It does not want to take up space in the world or be seen, and it subordinates itself to everyone and everything. It cannot imagine feeling other than inferior (although, in fact, it actually feels superior to individuals who feel superior!).

Inferiority and superiority are experiences of frightened parts of your personality. Some situations activate frightened parts of your personality that feel inferior, and others stimulate frightened parts of your personality that feel superior. For example, when you put someone on a pedestal (idolize her) you feel inferior to that person, but when she fails to meet your expectations (this always happens) she falls off the pedestal (you feel superior to her). The idol and pedestal are your creations. When you see your idol as a person like you, one illusion (you are inferior) disappears and another illusion (you are superior) replaces it. On the other hand, if you discover that someone you did not consider important (for example, a homeless person) can be very helpful to you (he is actually an eccentric billionaire), the reverse happens. The illusion that you are superior (he does not warrant your attention) is replaced by the illusion that you are inferior (your attention is drawn to him magnetically).

I was wearing work clothes while speaking with a contractor who was helping Linda and me improve our beautiful new home when a subcontractor walked up and abruptly interrupted me to speak with the contractor. When the contractor introduced me as the "property owner," his behavior suddenly and dramatically changed. He turned his full attention toward me, smiled charmingly, and extended his hand. Disregard turned into deference; one frightened part of his personality replaced another when he discovered that I was a potential employer instead of a laborer. He did not think in terms of frightened parts of the personality, but frightened parts of his personality shaped his perception and behavior first one way and then another.

Sometimes when I meet someone who has something I want, or I think can help me get what I want, I find myself engaging that person more than others, being more friendly, more available, and more interested in him or her. The tray I am on goes down, and the tray that person is on goes up. I feel inferior and I look up to him or her. The opposite also happens. Sometimes when I meet someone I think cannot help me in any way, I find myself less interested in that person, less available, and more distant in general. The tray I am on goes up, and the tray that person is on goes down. I look down on him or her. I feel superior. In the first case, I usually see things about the person that I admire (judge her positively), and in the second case I often see things about the person that I do not like or approve (judge her negatively). In both cases, I fail to see him or her as a soul.

These are experiences of inequality. In other words, they occur only when frightened parts of my personality are active. Frightened parts of the personality assess the external power of others and compare it with their own. When a frightened part of your personality calculates that it has more external power (ability to manipulate and control), you feel safe and valuable (superior), and your tray rises. When it calculates that it has less, you feel threatened and less valuable (inferior), and your tray sinks.

Feeling superior or feeling inferior is a message to you that a frightened part of your personality is active and determining your sensations, thoughts, perceptions, and intentions. Your scale (if you are picturing it) reflects this. Feeling inferior and feeling superior are red lights. They are signals to stop, take time to consider what a frightened part of your personality that feels superior (or a frightened part of your personality that feels inferior) has created in the past, and ask yourself if you want to create it again. How many collisions do you want to experience before you learn to recognize a red light?

Sometimes an individual who habitually feels inferior thinks that she is challenging her inferiority, but she is actually experiencing it in a different way. For example, a pleaser who never expresses how resentful and angry she feels when her attempts to please are not appreciated and decides to "set my boundaries" (no more pleasing) has not healed that frightened part of her personality. She has flipped from one end of it to the other, so to speak, from feeling inferior and needing to please to feeling superior and righteously angry. You cannot experience equality when a frightened part of your personality controls you.

Sometimes individuals create a false sense of humility by thinking of themselves as less than others, or below others. "Humility" of this type is superiority. It is not humble and it is not equality. Once a rabbi, a story goes, praying alone in the temple, glimpsed the infinitude of the Universe. Ritualistically tearing his shirt, he shouted in awe, "I am nobody! I am nobody!"

The chairman of the temple saw the rabbi in ecstasy and also tore his shirt and began to shout, "I am nobody!" The janitor, seeing the rabbi and the chairman, was also engulfed in ecstasy, tore his shirt, and exclaimed joyfully, "I am nobody! I am nobody!" At that, the chairman and rabbi fell silent. The chairman pointed to the janitor and said, "Look who thinks he's nobody."

Equality is a delightful experience. When the trays of your scale are level you walk in a friendly world. You enjoy people, and they enjoy you. Fellow travelers surround you and share the journey toward wholeness. You may feel equal with others, but unless you are free from thoughts of better or worse, or more or less (for example, beautiful, intelligent, worthy, wealthy, strong, talented, etc.), you are not equal.

When you are equal you are open, appreciative, relaxed, and comfortable. You share easily without second agendas, laugh easily, and are present. When you are not equal you are superior or inferior (frightened parts of your personality are active) and you feel distance from others, your interactions are forced or formal, and you judge and blame others or yourself. Whatever you do has a second agenda (external power).

When I was an army officer on Okinawa I spent most of my free time, like my peers, in the junior officer's club, where officers drank with officers of the same rank. Second lieutenants drank with second lieutenants, first lieutenants drank with first lieutenants, captains drank with captains, and so on. One evening a captain joined our table of second lieutenants and asked us to call him Irv (instead of Captain). We were uncomfortable (we felt inferior), but I could see that Irv was comfortable (he felt equal). After a while I asked him, "Why are you drinking with second lieutenants?" "I decided long ago not to let rank keep me from enjoying my companions in the army," he replied. I did not feel equal to Irv (on my scale, my tray was lower than Irv's tray), but Irv felt equal to me (on his scale, our trays were level).

I experienced another example of equality many years later

on Hawaii. A friend took Linda and me to meet his teacher, Auntie Margaret, a legendary Hawaiian healer. Her house was a center of activity and filled with students from many countries. I felt comfortable with her at once, with her toughness, knowledge of ancient Hawaiian healing, and huge heart. Shortly afterward, another friend took us to a beautiful remote beach. We noticed several Hawaiians in the distance, and soon a scowling woman approached angrily. "This is private property!" she proclaimed. "You have no right to be here." We apologized (even though the beach was public), but she left as disgruntled as she came. She was Auntie Margaret's (and Irv's) opposite. There was nothing I could do to open her heart, and there was nothing I could do to close Auntie Margaret's. Auntie Margaret (and Irv) felt equal (loving parts of the personality), and the angry woman felt superior (frightened parts of the personality).

Your scale does not compare or even register characteristics of personalities. It shows you whether you are relating to a personality or to a soul. All personalities are unique, and so none are equal. Some are strong and some are weak, some are young and some are old, some are wealthy and some are poor, and so on. When you perceive an individual as a personality, your tray rises or falls. When you perceive an individual as a soul, the trays on your scale are level.

You cannot be almost equal. The difference between equality and inequality is the difference between love and fear. When a frightened part of your personality assesses the external power of other personalities, your tray rises or sinks. Loving parts of your personality do not judge, and your scale is balanced.

Equality is the perception that nothing in the Universe is more precious than you and nothing in the Universe is less precious than you. Spiritual partnerships require it, and spiritual partners help one another develop it.

13

Dynamic 1

Growing Together

The dynamics of spiritual partnership are unlike the dynamics of any other relationship. Even the most dramatic images of difference—such as day-night, light-darkness, life-death—cannot convey the freshness, power, and potential of spiritual partnerships. These images depict completion and rebirth. As powerful as they are, they are inadequate to illuminate the depth, scope, and purpose of spiritual partnerships. Spiritual partnerships, along with multisensory perception and the new understandings and awareness that it brings, are not reborn experiences. They are appearing for the first time throughout the collective human consciousness. Spiritual partnership is a relationship archetype unlike any in our history.

Spiritual partners are colleagues, but not in the way that five-sensory individuals are colleagues. Just as students learning the same subject help one another with their homework, spiritual partners help one another with their life's work—spiritual growth. What one does not see in herself, others might. Eventually each sees in herself what she needs to change or cultivate in order to create a life of harmony, cooperation, sharing, and reverence for Life. Hungry individuals crave food. Spiritual partners crave meaning. They explore together what it is and how to create it. They observe what attracts them and what repulses them, what keeps them separate and what connects them, and they help one another to grow spiritually.

For example, my mother idolized me. I was exempt from her

criticism and was the constant recipient of her admiration. Her adoration softened, rationalized, and made acceptable to her whatever I did. I grew up without recognizing the difference between her love for me and the pedestal she built for me. I am not sure that she distinguished between them before she left the Earth school, but my experiences of her adoration influenced my interactions with Linda again and again.

I became angry when I felt that Linda did not listen to me attentively or replied absentmindedly, and I blamed her for my anger. There is a big difference between holding a person or circumstance responsible for your emotional pain and recognizing a frightened part of your personality as the cause of it. In the first case, you need to change someone or something outside of you in order to relieve your pain. In the second case, you need to change yourself in order to eliminate it. This is the difference between reacting and responding; creating with fear and creating with love; pursuing external power and creating authentic power. It is also the difference between wielding your creative power irresponsibly (unconsciously) and using it responsibly (consciously).

Each time I blamed Linda for my anger I distracted myself from the pain that generated it, and a frightened part of my personality went unnoticed (by me) and unchallenged. When that part of my personality was triggered again (by Linda, for example), I became angry again. Recognizing the relationship between my anger when Linda did not adore me (listen to me like a fascinated puppy) and my mother's adoration did not prevent my anger from recurring. Discussing it with Linda did not prevent my anger from recurring. No analysis could uproot my anger. When I felt that Linda failed to listen to me, I became angry.

When Linda and I began our journey together, my need to be adored in order to feel safe and valuable interlocked perfectly with her need to be in a relationship with a man in order to feel safe and valuable. This complementary interaction between frightened parts of my personality and frightened parts of hers was our honeymoon, a prelude to potential intimacy. All relationships have one. Then the partners begin to see one another more as they are and less as they would like one another to be. Like grass growing through cracks in a sidewalk, previously unnoticed behaviors become visible. For example, one partner needs to dominate (such as I did), and another needs to please (such as Linda did), etc.

This ends the honeymoon. Fantasies of effortless fulfillment are replaced by interactions between real and complex personalities. When illusory perceptions dissolve, individuals in an old-type relationship think that their relationship is failing, and they focus on "saving" it. They get therapy, explore their stories, ask for advice, or just try to get along better. If all else fails they settle for a painful relationship that fulfills neither of them but helps each feel secure, or they separate.

When fantasies of effortless fulfillment dissolve in a spiritual partnership, a spiritual partner challenges the frightened parts of his or her personality that react to real and complex personalities. In short, individuals in old-type relationships attempt to change one another (pursue external power). Spiritual partners change themselves (create authentic power). If Linda or I, for example, had not chosen to use our painful emotional experiences to grow spiritually, we could not have developed or deepened a spiritual partnership. We used tools that individuals in old-type relationships do not have.

We applied emotional awareness when we were upset—scanning for physical sensations in our bodies that tell us when a frightened part of the personality is active (they are painful) and when a loving part is active (they feel good). We noticed our thoughts that tell us when a frightened part of the personality is active (they are judgmental, critical, etc.) and when a loving part is active (they are thoughts of gratitude, appreciation, care, etc.). If my thoughts were judgmental, violent, or addictively sexual, for example, I knew that a frightened part of my personality was active. We examined our intentions that tell us when a frightened part of the personality is active (it intends to win, to be right, to control—in other words, to pursue external power), and when a loving part is active (it intends to create harmony, cooperate, share, and revere Life). If my intention was to dominate, to be right, or to prove Linda wrong, for example, I knew that a frightened part of my personality was active. Then I chose an intention to create a constructive consequence instead of the destructive consequences that I knew the intention of the frightened part of my personality would create (this is a responsible choice).

I chose to listen, for example, instead of speak; to understand instead of demand to be understood; to be patient instead of hurried, and so on. Whatever I chose, it was different and often opposite from what the frightened part of my personality would have chosen (and wanted very much to do in that moment)—such as justify myself, explain myself, shut Linda off, hurry through our interaction, withdraw, or shout. Linda did the same. As our spiritual partnership developed, I realized that my interactions with Linda were changing me in ways that I had always wanted. It took discipline that I did not know I had—and often didn't—but I was determined to change everything in myself that had caused me so much pain and loneliness, along with everything that I didn't like when I saw it in others. Linda did the same.

Experiencing the full force of a frightened part of the personality instead of shouting (or withdrawing emotionally, eating, shopping, watching pornography, gambling, etc.) is very difficult. Spiritual partners support one another in experiencing their emotions (frightened and loving parts of their personalities), and while they are experiencing their emotions they make choices that will create the most constructive consequences possible. That is how I came to terms (and continue to come to terms) with the frightened part of my personality that demands adoration. I experience the painful physical sensations of a frightened part of my personality when I am ignored (or think that I am ignored), and at the same time I choose a response to that pain (instead of the reaction that the frightened part of my personality always chooses).

If I had succeeded in manipulating Linda with my anger into a prolonged pretense of adoration, I would still be in the control of a frightened part of my personality that demands adoration and she would still pretend to adore me. She would also resent me for manipulating her and resent herself for allowing the manipulation—for distorting her life to avoid my reactions and her fear of loneliness rather than creating a healthy life. I chose to examine carefully (experience fully) my emotions when Linda did not adore me and respond instead of react, and she supported me in doing this. Linda chose to examine carefully her emotions when I did not appear to be pleased by her and chose to respond instead of react, and I supported her.

Sometimes I am able to create authentic power while Linda is reacting instead of responding (for example, is angry, feels overwhelmed, needs to please, or fears abandonment), and sometimes Linda creates authentic power while I am reacting (for example, making things more important than people; thinking of myself first and others next, if at all; or feeling (and acting) entitled). My creating authentic power does not have to do with what Linda chooses in the moment, and her creating authentic power does not have to do with what I choose.

Spiritual partners are not satisfied with stagnant or destructive relationships, no matter how familiar or enduring they are. They are not content to remain on the treadmill of satisfying the needs of frightened parts of the personality. For example, when a spiritual partner becomes defensive ("What does it matter if I ate the chocolate!"), her partners will bring that frightened part of her personality to her attention. They will inquire about her intention. They will remind her to look for physical sensations in certain parts of her body and help her to challenge frightened parts of her personality and cultivate loving parts.*

Spiritual partners ask themselves which of their activities create authentic power and which pursue external power, and choose to create authentic power. When they forget that they are together in order to grow spiritually, they recommit to growing spiritually when they remember. Children, lifestyles, hairstyles, purchases, education, work, and all else take on different meaning for them. They distinguish endeavors that originate in love from those that originate in fear, and choose those that originate in love. If they find themselves seeking recognition, influence, or approval in order to feel safe and valuable, they change their intention. They are not content to navigate inland waterways. They sail courageously on the open ocean.

Few individuals have plumbed the depths of their rage, hatred, terror, jealousy, and despair or the scope of their wisdom and power of their compassion, yet these currents run beneath the surface of awareness in each of us, like great rivers on the floor of an ocean. Spiritual partners help one another discover and explore them. Spiritual partners give one another permission to experience frightened parts of their personalities and heal them and loving parts of their personalities and cultivate them. They are fellow travelers bound for the same destination, each responsible for the journey, and each committed to completing it.

The more spiritual partners challenge frightened parts of their personalities, the more they are able to support one another, the more creativity they have to share, and the more fulfilled they become. For example, Linda and I were once in a power struggle trying to plan a new event. We mistook questions for accusa-

---

* Challenging frightened parts of your personality and cultivating loving parts of your personality require *responsible choice* in addition to emotional awareness. To learn more about responsible choice, I recommend *The Mind of the Soul: Responsible Choice* (Gary Zukav and Linda Francis, Simon & Schuster, 2003). It shows you step-by-step how to make responsible choices and practice choosing responsibly. (Be sure to do the exercises.)

tions and suggestions for criticisms. Each painful exchange triggered reactions in us. Frightened parts of my personality locked in competition with frightened parts of hers. At the end of the day we were fatigued, impatient, and annoyed—in the service of teaching authentic power!

When we realized how far we had traveled in a direction that we did not want to go, we decided to stop and start over. We reconnected. We set new intentions to cocreate. Linda modeled starting over for me, and I did my best to model it for her. If we had not been committed to growing spiritually, the power struggle would have raged on like a forest fire out of control. I could have ended it in me at any time (if I had remembered my commitment to growing spiritually—but I didn't), and Linda could have ended it in her (if she had remembered her commitment). In this case, we ended it together, and the event that we cocreated reflected this healthy process. It was fresh, deep, and joyful.

There is no security in a spiritual partnership. Spiritual partners are together to grow spiritually, not soothe one another's fears. On the contrary, they support one another in experiencing their fears and healing the sources of them. Spiritual partners are patient and caring, but patience and care are not enough to keep them together. They appreciate one another, but appreciation is not enough either. They love one another, but even love is not enough. Only commitment to creating authentic power can keep spiritual partners together through the challenges of unearthing, experiencing, and healing frightened parts of their personalities. Five-sensory individuals in old-type relationships commit to one another, their relationships, and their five-sensory goals. Spiritual partners commit to growing spiritually and to supporting one another in growing spiritually.

Frightened parts of your personality do not threaten a spiritual partnership, but failing to challenge them does. Each time you challenge a frightened part of your personality it reasserts itself, offering you more opportunities to challenge and heal it until it disappears (this is how authentic power is created). Getting stuck in a frightened part of your personality does not threaten a spiritual partnership either, but staying stuck does. If a spiritual partner refuses again and again to budge from his or her angry, defensive, withdrawn, or vengeful experiences ("Leave me alone!" "I don't want to hear this anymore." "This is the way that I am and I don't want to change!"), the reason for the spiritual partnership (spiritual growth) disappears. It is one thing to get caught in a frightened part of your personality. Spiritual partnerships provide you opportunities to experience the frightened parts of your personality and getting caught in one, sometimes repeatedly, is part of the experience of growing spiritually. It is another thing to refuse again and again to challenge a frightened part of your personality (such as your anger, jealousy, or vengefulness). When the reason for a spiritual partnership ceases to exist, so does the partnership.

Spiritual partners recognize themselves as equals in partnership for the purpose of spiritual growth. Five-sensory individuals in old-type relationships do not have this perspective. They enter and leave relationships as necessary for their sense of security and value. They blame one another for their distress and happiness, and they stay together as long as they assist one another to survive or enhance their comfort.

Spiritual partners stay together as long as they grow together. That is the first dynamic of spiritual partnership.

14

Dynamic 2

Choosing Roles

When an actor assumes a role he leaves all thoughts, feelings, and intentions aside except those that belong to the character he is playing. He sees through the eyes of that character, hears through its ears, longs for what the character wants, takes comfort in what the character achieves, and is distressed at what the character fails to achieve. His life is not his while he is on the stage. It belongs to the role that he is playing. He cannot break character; above all else he must be true to the character. The more true to his character he becomes, the more real the character becomes to the audience, and the more the play comes to life. Outside the theater he can be himself again, but onstage only the role of his character exists. Even while he waits in the wings for his cue he stays in the role of his character. Sometimes an actor becomes so involved in his role that he remains in character between acts. If an actor becomes compulsively involved in the life of his character, he lives that role wherever he goes. This is not healthy.

Most people, like the obsessive actor, live the life of the character they are playing wherever they go although they are not aware of playing a role. They never break character, even when they are alone. They remain in their role when they are with friends and family, when they drive and shower, when they eat and work. For example, the role of Mother is the dominant role for many women, even if they have careers, although many women who have children play the role of Businessperson, Athlete,

Teacher, and so on. Each individual plays many roles, and whatever the role is, it defines her perceptions, thoughts, experiences, and intentions while she is playing it. The more involved in a role an individual becomes, the less aware of her role she is—in other words, the more invisible (unconscious) it is to her.

Roles determine how we interact. I played the role of a manly, sexual, rebellious, disdainful Adventurer for many years, and all the while I was unknowingly confined by that role. The role had nothing to do with how other people experienced me, but it did determine how I experienced myself. For example, the role did not allow me to express (or even experience) confusion, helplessness, or emotional pain. Grief and tears were out of character. On the other hand, anger, smoking, drinking, recklessness, and disregard for others were acceptable. Intelligence, creativity, and concern for me were OK, too, but not tenderness or care for others. Individuals who were not attracted to my role saw me more accurately as an angry, addicted, narcissistic sexual predator and avoided me. Little, if anything, about my role was acceptable to their roles.

Roles attract roles. Artists attract Artists, for example, and within that role subroles such as Musician, Sculptor, Painter, Writer, and Poet attract one another. Everyone plays many roles during a lifetime and several of them simultaneously, such as Father, Businessman, and Golfer (a subrole of the role of Athlete); or Mother, Wife, and Teacher; or Politician and Mother; and so on. An individual who can see himself in only one role is analogous to an obsessive actor who cannot leave his stage role behind. He is lost in it. His friends forget who he is without the role, his family forgets who he is without the role, and eventually he forgets who he is without the role.

Identification with an illness creates a role of Sick Person that changes behavior and limits creativity. Without identification the same illness could provide opportunities to expand consciousness, create new behaviors, surpass previous limitations, and unleash creativity. "Misfortunes" such as bankruptcy, business failure, and the death of a spouse or child can also create roles. Even commitment to growing spiritually can become disfigured into the role of Spiritual Person. A role temporarily anesthetizes the pain of powerlessness. For example, the more you identify yourself as a Mother, Businessperson, Professional, Adventurer, Spiritual Person, etc., the more you attempt to manipulate and control others with it and the more you mask the pain of powerlessness.

Before I did a series of television shows with Oprah Winfrey my role was superior backcountry Recluse. Afterward my role became Celebrity. This was a new role for me, but it was just as confining as my previous role. Earlier I played the roles of Student and then Soldier (which were compatible with my role of manly, sexual, rebellious Adventurer). Playing a role does not mean choosing one as you might for a high school play and then practicing, refining, and presenting it on opening night. It is being captured by a self-perception and internal experiences that seem so natural, even if they are painful, that you cannot imagine being any other way.

Roles that you play to avoid your feelings, potential, and responsibility are unnecessary, draining, and exploitative. Like stage sets that appear attractive to the audience but are held crudely in place from behind, roles are facades. When roles cease to control you, you become able to choose them and use them. Roles that choose you (that seem so natural that you cannot imagine being another way) imprison you. Roles that you choose are vehicles to express your love. Like a musician who plays the flute, cello, and piano, you choose the instrument to fit your need; the appropriate role allows you to give your gifts in the moment. If a role originates in love, ceasing to see yourself in it will have no effect upon your sense of security and self-worth. If a role originates in fear, you will feel vulnerable, disoriented, and lost without it.

Imagine what your life would be if you no longer had a familiar role to play, for example, Mother (or Businessperson, Educator, Craftsperson, etc.). This does not mean ceasing to be a mother. It means ceasing to identify yourself as a Mother, view yourself as a Mother, and experience yourself as a Mother and experiment instead with experiencing yourself as a personality with frightened and loving parts and, at the same time, an immortal soul. It means ceasing to use the role of Mother to shield you from frightening experiences such as attention from men, career demands, feelings of worthlessness, and insecurity.

Individuals who are not aware of the roles that imprison them are not aware of choosing them. They are like individuals who do not recognize that their reactions, such as shouting and emotional withdrawal, are choices. Once they become aware of their roles as ways of manipulating and controlling others, they are free of the constraints of those roles, just as individuals who become aware that their reactions are choices acquire the ability to respond. They are also free to change their roles and choose other roles.

For example, when I became a grandfather I was surprised by new experiences. I felt that I was suddenly a different person in some ways. The role of Grandfather required that I love my grandchildren more than other children, which I did. However, I questioned whether I wanted to love some souls who were beginning a journey through the Earth school more than others. I also realized that I felt safer, more important, and more worthy when I loved my grandchildren more than other children, although I did not know why. (This is an experience of a role choosing you. You enter the influence of an energy archetype without recognizing it, and that archetype shapes your perceptions and experiences.) The change I needed to make in myself, I realized, was not to love my grandchildren less but to love other children more. Slowly a new experience of Grandfather developed for me. (This is an experience of transforming an energy archetype through conscious participation in it.) As a result, the role ceased to control me and I began to use it. Eventually I began to see all children as my grandchildren.

This is the difference between the experiences of an unconscious role (I love my grandchildren more than all other children) and the experiences of a conscious role (all children are my grandchildren). It is also the difference between the experiences of the unconscious role of Businessperson (I sell goods and services to maximize revenue and profit) and the experiences of the conscious role of Businessperson (I sell goods and services to support individuals in healthy, wise, and compassionate ways); the experiences of the unconscious role of Athlete (I compete to win and be recognized) and the experiences of the conscious role of Athlete (I test my strength and skill against others to reach my fullest potential); and so on.

Roles that we do not always notice but that shape our experiences strongly are those associated with gender (man, woman), race (white, yellow, black, red), and nationality (American, Japanese, Mexican, etc.). They are powerful, often invisible, and they take control of the personality without notice. For example, the natural affinity for one another of individuals who play the role of Father (which includes subroles such as American Father and Iraqi Father) was eclipsed when young men playing the role of Muslim Avenger killed thousands of fathers and children of fathers in the World Trade Center and the Pentagon. Then thousands of individuals playing the role of American Avenger killed thousands more fathers and children of fathers. (The role of Avenger has many subroles, such as Christian Avenger, Hindu Avenger, Jewish Avenger, Palestinian Avenger, and Black, Brown, Red, and Yellow Avenger, to name a few.)

A role is an energy archetype, or template, such as Mother, Father, Student, Artist, and so on. When you step into a role, such as Wife or Husband, you enter the energy sphere of that template, or archetype. You fall into its gravitational pull, so to speak, like a moon orbiting a planet. Couples who enjoyed themselves as single friends, for example, discover that their relationship changes when they marry. Stresses that were not present before become part of their experience. They invoked the archetypes of Marriage, Husband, and Wife by marrying, and those archetypes began to define their experiences.

If an individual is unaware of his identification with a role (uses it unthinkingly to feel safe and valuable), the role increasingly influences his experiences. He interacts with others as a Husband, for example, and his perceptions and experiences are shaped by his participation in the archetypes of Husband and Marriage. He sees from those perspectives, and they are different from the perspectives of other archetypes.

I excelled at debate in high school. It didn't matter to me whether I argued for or against a proposition. Only winning mattered. Losing a round, much less a tournament, was extremely painful. I didn't know about the pursuit of external power or frightened parts of my personality, but I experienced both. Later in my life, when I looked back at my successes in debate and elsewhere, they felt so empty that I determined to never again use my speaking abilities to manipulate or control. As a result, my public talks, when I began to give them, were as lifeless and monotone as my interactions with others had become. It did not occur to me that I could use the same abilities that I had previously used to win debate tournaments in order to feel safe and valuable to share about authentic power without attachment to the outcome.

In my determination to be authentic ("who I really am") I imprisoned myself for decades in the role of serious, deep, caring (and humorless) Teacher. This role prevented me from sharing about authentic power in the most effective ways (and enjoying myself). I did not realize that I had chosen this role and that I could choose other roles to help me explain authentic power (and enjoy myself).

Five-sensory individuals play the role of Human Living on the Earth. Multisensory perception provides each of us the accurate self-perception of a powerful and creative, compassionate and loving spirit instead. This perception is not a role. It is freedom from roles. It also offers spiritual partnership—partnership among equals for the purpose of spiritual growth—as a vehicle for souls voluntarily learning lessons of power, wisdom, responsibility, and love in the arena of the five senses to support one another in creating authentic power.

When an individual brings spiritual partnership into his marriage, he participates in the evolution of the archetype of Marriage into the archetype of Spiritual Partnership. This is happening in millions of marriages. The limitations (emotional reactions and unconsciously chosen intentions) and requirements (external power) of five-sensory Husbands and Wives are being replaced with the larger capacities (emotional awareness and responsible choice) and different potential (authentic power) of multisensory humans. When you choose the role of Spiritual Partner, you bring the perception of power as the alignment of your personality with your soul into all of your roles.

Culture and custom dictate the roles of five-sensory humans (frightened parts of the personality choose acceptable roles). Multisensory individuals are not confined to traditional roles. Multisensory males can choose to be stay-at-home fathers, executives, carpenters, or nurses, and multisensory females can choose to work in construction, as professionals, and in boardrooms. The full range of human activity is available to them, limited only by their aptitudes and interests. Multisensory humans also develop new roles to access their creativity, deepen their fulfillment, and enrich their lives—roles such as Friend of All, Celebrator of Life, Cocreator with Life, Cocreator with the Earth, and more.

The more you create authentic power, the less frightened parts of your personality choose your roles unconsciously, the more loving parts of your personality choose them consciously, and the more you contribute to your well-being and the well-being of the collectives in which you participate. The most inclusive collective is Life. Therefore, the role that will eventually call to all of us is Universal Human. A Universal Human is beyond nation, culture, religion, race, and sex. A Universal Human is a citizen of the Universe whose allegiance is to Life first and all else second. All roles are subroles of the Universal Human. A Universal Human is a part of Life first and an American second; a part of Life first and a male second; a part of Life first and a Mother/Father/Christian/Jew/Muslim/Hindu and so on second. A musician who plays many different instruments does not play them because she loves instruments. She plays them because she loves music. A Universal Human does not love roles. She loves Life.

When you align your personality with your soul, you do not acquire another, larger identity for your fears to exploit. You remove the sources of your fears. When you create authentic power and support others in growing spiritually, you choose your roles with the healthiest parts of your personality. When others do the same thing, they choose their roles, too, with the healthiest parts of their personalities.

Spiritual partners choose their roles.

That is the second dynamic of spiritual partnership.

15

Dynamic 3
Saying What Is Most Difficult

Five-sensory humans in old-type relationships conceal the things they are most frightened will destroy their relationship. Spiritual partners share the things they are most frightened will destroy their partnership. This is the third dynamic of spiritual partnership.

Spiritual partners know that not sharing what they are most frightened to share is like burying dynamite. A wall forms when a spiritual partner hides a secret that he fears will end his partnership. It cannot be climbed, burrowed under, tunneled through, or broken down. Impenetrable and invisible, it prevents or destroys intimacy. The one who keeps the secret does not trust his partners, and they feel it.

The burden of the secret grows heavier with time. It requires constant vigilance lest a clue, or the secret itself, be inadvertently revealed. It haunts the holder, an unseen and relentless tormentor. Fear of revealing the secret and pain of keeping it combine to isolate the one with the secret from his spiritual partners. It stands between them like a cloud blocking the sun.

Eventually, the secret distorts every thought and action. The relationship that it threatens becomes corrupt in the keeping. Trust slowly and painfully vanishes. The secret might not be as destructive to others as the one who keeps it fears, but his efforts to hide it and growing fear of revealing it make sharing it more and more difficult. As long as the secret is held, the partnership cannot function as it was designed to function. The secret may be abuse of a child, abuse as a child, committing a crime or wanting to, wishing ill for another or celebrating it, infidelity or suspicion of it. Whatever the secret, it becomes increasingly painful to ponder, shameful to remember, and terrifying to share. At last the dynamite explodes.

Secrets kept in fear are burdens. Secrets kept in love are not. For example, keeping the secret of a same-sex attraction from those who might disapprove is an exhausting experience. Keeping the secret of a surprise birthday party is a delight. The first secret is kept by frightened parts of the personality and the second by loving parts of the personality. If the party is discovered, no one feels ashamed or uncomfortable. No relationships are threatened. They are deepened. The love that created the secret is revealed along with the secret.

When fear motivates a secret, a facade replaces authenticity, falsehood replaces honesty, and deceit replaces integrity. Spontaneity diminishes and then dies. Creativity depletes the keeper of the secret rather than refreshes her, for example, devising false explanations for previous false explanations. Whatever you feel that you should not be and know that you are—or want to be—is your secret, and keeping it confines you. Whether your family expects you to love business and you love music, you are a woman attracted to women or a man attracted to men, you are generous when you are expected to be frugal, or you feel jealousy, rage, or despair and you feel that you should not—moving beyond your fear with the intention to heal moves you toward health. Remaining bound by your fear keeps you from it.

Until you can say what is most difficult for you to say, you cannot speak from your heart, live unafraid, create health, or receive support from others. Sharing a secret in fear (with the intention to manipulate and control) is the same as keeping a secret in fear (with the intention to manipulate and control). You do not challenge frightened parts of your personality, and they continue to create destructive consequences. When you share a secret with the intention to create authentic power you move toward wholeness, new possibilities appear, and your fear does not control you. You cultivate a loving part of your personality and challenge a frightened part. You become who you are instead of who others expect you to be, or who you think they expect you to be.

In 1948 two brothers discovered an earthenware jar buried in the desert near Nag Hammadi in Upper Egypt. It contained thirteen papyrus books bound in leather. They took the books home where their mother used many of the pages for tinder. Scholars later realized, with great excitement, that the books were created by very early Christians who are now called gnostics (nos tiks) (from the Greek word *gnōsis,* which is usually translated—in reference to these early Christians—as "insight"). The church declared the gnostics heretics in the second century AD. Fleeing fellow Christians, torture, and death, they hid their books where the brothers found them seventeen hundred years later.

These books have become known as the gnostic gospels. They are not the same as the gospels in hotel-room bibles. In fact, they are not mentioned by the modern church or found in its literature, yet they appear to scholars to be authentic. They paint a picture of Christ and Christianity that is very different from the picture that commonly available gospels paint. For example, gnostic Christians included women in the priesthood, believed in reincarnation, and taught that intermediaries between us and God (priests) were unnecessary. These beliefs and practices, among others, made the gnostics (very) unpopular with the church that we recognize today.

Like the biblical gospels, the gnostic gospels purport to describe words and actions of Christ. My favorite is the Gospel of Thomas. According to it, Christ said:

> If you bring forth what is within you,
> What you bring forth will save you.
> If you do not bring forth what is within you,
> What you do not bring forth will destroy you.

If you do not bring forth the truth of your heart, how can you give the gifts that you were born to give? How can you create the life that is waiting for you while you are frightened to tell your parents about it, or your boss that you are quitting your job as a banker to become a gardener? How can you leave the children with your husband while you study medicine, or quit your tenured position to be with your children? How can you walk comfortably in the world when you fear that others will discover what you are, what you think, and how you want to live?

Several years after I left the army I became intermittently depressed, but I feared to share my pain—first because I feared I could not express it, then because I feared no one could understand it, then because I feared others would judge me, and then because I feared to impose my pain on them. These were my reasons for not sharing, but I did not think about my deeper intentions for not sharing. I did not think about intentions at all. Each painful spiral downward into isolation made asking for help more difficult until it became impossible. These are experiences of frightened parts of the personality. I did not value myself, and I could not imagine others valuing me (this is the pain of powerlessness). I did not know how many more episodes of the pain I could endure. I felt like a black hole, and, energetically, I was.

A seed that cannot break through the surface of compacted soil curls back upon its distorted self and dies. In the same way, potential that cannot break through encrusted fear becomes frustration, resentment, hopelessness, anger, and rage. Self-hatred is self-destruction. Remaining less than you need to be cultivates frightened parts of your personality instead of loving parts, and they grow stronger. Keeping a secret in fear is the choice of isolation and confinement instead of intimacy and freedom. The secret prevents the seed from sprouting, the plant from growing, and the flower from blooming. You are the seed, the plant is your life, and the blossom is authentic power.

While I was struggling with depression, addicted to sex, and frightened about my rent, a friend invited me to a weekly meeting of physicists at the Lawrence Berkeley Laboratory. (I was living in San Francisco.) I did not realize it at the time, but my life began to change at that meeting. I was fascinated with the discussion I overheard ("Do we create the reality that we experiment with?"). Afterward I could think of nothing but the meeting. I began to read about quantum physics and question my new physicist friends about it. The more I understood the fundamental concepts, the more excited I became; and the more excited I became, the more I wanted to share them. When the idea to write a book about quantum physics for nonscientists like me came, it felt natural and appropriate, even though I had never written a book or studied science.

I wrote the book as a gift to those who would come after me with an interest in quantum physics. I wanted to give them "on a silver platter" everything that I had learned, including the fruits of many tutorials that gracious physicists were giving to me. As the book expanded, so did I. Nothing in my life to that time was as engaging, enjoyable, and fulfilling as writing it. The day before the book was published, a wonderful review of it appeared in *The New York Times*. It soon won numerous awards and was translated into many languages. I intended to make quantum mechanics understandable to as many people as I could so that they could apply its empowering concepts to their lives and as many disciplines as possible, and I did. The whole experience was purely wonderful.

My experiences before, during, and after writing the book illustrate for me my favorite excerpt from the Gospel of Thomas. What I was not bringing forth while I was searching for sex, riding motorcycles, experimenting with drugs, and proving my manliness was destroying me, but I did not recognize it. Krishna tells a hero of the Mahabharata, the epic poem of Hinduism, "Destruction never approaches weapon in hand. It comes slyly on tiptoe, making you see bad in good and good in bad." I took pride in what I was and what I did even while depression and anger increasingly corroded my life. Destruction on tiptoe had arrived.

All of these painful experiences—anger, jealousy, depression, need for sex, and terror at not being able to pay the rent—disappeared when I was writing the book. I brought forth my first gift to Life and changed my life in the process. Writing my book required a decision, although in this case it was an easy decision. I was not aware of the choices I had made that led to the hell of depression and rage, but I was aware of the choice that I made to give others the gifts that were being given to me, and that choice made all the difference.

Spiritual partners are multisensory. They often know the secret that you withhold, and they know why you withhold it (a frightened part of your personality is active, and you are not challenging it). "Are you attracted to that woman in green?" Linda asked me while we danced during one of our first evenings out together. I was embarrassed because Linda had seen what I had hoped was invisible—the intention of a frightened part of my personality to prey upon a fellow student in the Earth school. I was frightened because I wanted to cultivate our new partnership, not end it that evening. The frightened part of my personality intended to feel safe and valuable by seducing a woman. I intended to challenge it and continue to challenge it until it no longer tormented me.

I did not know how to explain that to Linda—that a frightened part of my personality wanted one thing, loving parts wanted another, and I intended to create with the loving parts. In the meanwhile, I felt my attraction, my embarrassment, and my fear. "Yes," I said. Linda was not angry. Perhaps she was challenging frightened parts of her personality, but she looked at me with appreciation. "I know," she told me. "I have never been with a man who answered honestly when I asked about what I already knew."

A dishonest answer would have placed our new partnership, in Linda's eyes, in the category of unsatisfactory relationships that she intended to avoid. "This is a new experience for me," she continued. "I am amazed by it."

Fulfilling and amazing experiences await spiritual partners as they support one another in challenging and healing frightened parts of their personalities and cultivating and strengthening loving parts of their personalities with courage and integrity. Five-sensory humans in old-type relationships focus on their secrets. Spiritual partners focus on challenging the frightened parts of their personalities that need secrets. Indulging frightened parts of your personality or challenging them is a choice. Keeping a secret in fear or sharing in love is the same choice.

When you move beyond the prison of a secret you attract individuals who no longer need secrets. You resonate with them as you previously resonated with individuals who fear to share what they think will destroy their relationships. Sharing what is most difficult with the intention to create authentic power requires clarity and appropriateness. For example, revealing your addiction to pornography to a store clerk would be inappropriate and counterproductive. Sharing with those who understand and support you (such as your spiritual partners) is often a good way to start. Your sharing can also be dramatic and public. The more you challenge frightened parts of your personality that fear sharing, the less you will fear others discovering what those parts want to keep secret.

Five-sensory humans keep secrets to manipulate one another. They guard their secrets, grow old with their secrets, and often die with their secrets. Spiritual partners share the things they most fear will destroy their partnership in order to create authentic power.

They intend to live and die in love.

16

Soul Summary

Anew type of human relationship is replacing every old-type relationship. This new type of relationship is designed for the new multisensory human who is creating authentic power.

SPIRITUAL PARTNERSHIPS—WHAT

- Spiritual partnership is partnership between equals for the purpose of spiritual growth.
- Friendships are not spiritual partnerships.
- Only spiritual partnerships can satisfy individuals who are creating authentic power.
- Individuals who are creating authentic power form spiritual partnerships with one another naturally.
- Spiritual partnership requires equality among all the partners.
- Each spiritual partner creates equality in himself or herself.
- Spiritual partners:
    Stay together as long as they grow together.
    Choose their own roles.
    Say the things they are most afraid will destroy their
        partnership.

Understanding spiritual partnerships allows you to recognize them, experiment with them, and appreciate them. They are different from any previous type of relationship, and so are the individuals who are drawn to them.

Understanding spiritual partnerships is not the same as experiencing spiritual partnership. As you create spiritual partnerships, benefits appear that you could not have imagined and the experience of them is healing, deep, and real.

17

Benefits of Spiritual Partnership

Commitment to creating authentic power is the prerequisite for a spiritual partnership. The benefit of a spiritual partnership is creating authentic power. The two come together. Authentic power and spiritual partnership are different facets of the same jewel. When the jewel (multisensory perception) came into being, so did its facets.

Creating authentic power is an interior process. Only you can become aware of your emotions, consult intuition, respond instead of react, and consciously shape energy into matter with your will. Growing from child to adult does not require will. Muscles and neurons grow, self-identity emerges, and conceptual understanding develops—all without your volition. Transforming yourself from unempowered to empowered is a different story. That requires aligning your personality with your soul, and aligning your personality with your soul requires will. Spiritual partners commit to aligning their personalities with their souls.

The benefits of spiritual partnership are as many as particles of sand on a beach—tenderness suddenly replacing rigidity and judgment, intimacy returning after a journey into despair, reawakening to meaning and awe, reverence replacing disdain, and countless other experiences of sanity and health replacing isolation and pain. Each is life-changing. In other words, spiritual partnerships provide spiritual partners countless opportunities to expand in love, experience grace, and create authentic power. Any list is partial at best, a group of road signs, each pointing toward more possible destinations. Wherever you are they appear, calling you always toward your highest potential, the life that you were born to live, and bliss.

The benefits of spiritual partnership are the highest goals that you can reach for, such as freedom from fear, and also the most grounded, pragmatic, and useful tools that you can develop, such as how to use power struggles to grow spiritually. All the benefits of spiritual partnership are interconnected, and each leads to others. Here are some.

- **Love for Yourself.** Love is a state of being. It is not an emotion or response. You cannot create Love, but you can experience it, and when you do it envelopes you. You cannot love one person or one thing more than another. Love makes all things precious, including you. It eliminates all constraints. Love is without limits, conditions, judgments, and hidden agendas. A flashlight can be turned off and on. The sun cannot be turned off. Confusing need with love is like confusing your flashlight with the sun. When you love, you and Love become indistinguishable, and love for others and love for you become indistinguishable.
- **Meaning and Purpose.** Traveling in the direction that your soul wants to go fills you with meaning. Traveling in other directions diminishes meaning in your life. Traveling in the opposite direction empties your life of meaning. The intentions of harmony, cooperation, sharing, and reverence for Life take you exactly where your soul wants to go—toward people, Life, health, fulfillment instead of satisfaction, and joy instead of happiness. Your life becomes worth living, and you become worthy of living it. These are experiences of authentic power.
- **Joy of Conscious Cocreation.** Every species and individual loves to play. Children play with grass, flowers, pets, food,

and one another. Theater ("plays"), music, movies, sports, and social interactions are forms of play. Creativity is play. Cocreation is the nectar of play. The less fear is present in your life, the more play is possible. When fear is absent, all is play. Athletes love the zone, musicians love the groove, and artists love the energy of the work because fear is absent there. As spiritual partners learn to cocreate without fear, their endeavors become play.

- **Real Courage.** Courage enables action when a frightened part of your personality is active. Some courageous actions are noble, such as risking injury to save another, and some are not, such as attempting to impress others (pursue external power) by doing something dangerous. Fear generates courage when you challenge frightened parts of your personality in order to be accepted, admired, or successful. Love generates courage when you challenge a frightened part of your personality in order to benefit another or to create authentic power. That is real courage. It takes courage to do dangerous things in order to prove yourself worthy (such as parachuting and combat patrols), but it takes ever so much more courage to challenge a frightened part of your personality that wants to shout, judge, resent, withdraw, or rage. Creating authentic power requires real courage. Spiritual partners help one another develop it.

- **Intimacy That Comes from Integrity.** Integrity is honoring the needs of the healthiest parts of your personality. Integrity is different from conscience. Conscience is the sense of what you *should* do in order to honor the expectations of your culture, peers, or family. If you do not "follow your conscience," you feel guilty. Integrity means wholeness. Living with integrity means acting with the healthiest parts of your personality, choosing loving intentions, and creating constructively even if you are frightened. Integrity opens the door to intimacy. Spiritual partners walk through it together.

- **Ability to Use Dramas and Tragedies to Grow Spiritually.** "Dramas" and "tragedies" are experiences of frightened parts of the personality. When you say, "What a tragedy this is!" you can more accurately say, "What a fear this is!" When you are immersed in a drama around you or within you, you can detach from it and recognize it as an experience of fear. Then apply the Spiritual Partnership Guidelines (next section)— scan your emotional energy system, consult intuition, and choose responsibly. Spiritual partners help one another do these things.

- **Deeper Commitment to Spiritual Growth.** Commitment is the foundation of spiritual growth. Without it you float on thoughts, wishes, desires, and ungrounded aspirations at best. At worst you are blown about by frightened parts of your personality like raindrops in a gale. Commitment to growing spiritually—creating authentic power—moves you into the driver's seat of your life. Without it you are taken for a ride to unpleasant places that are chosen by frightened parts of your personality. When you reach joyful destinations of your choosing that fulfill you in ways that you could not have imagined, the benefits of authentic power and spiritual partnerships become undeniable. You do not need to believe in them because you are living them. That is the way to discover that nothing is more important to you than growing spiritually.

- **Compassion for Yourself and Others.** If you are unable to distinguish between frightened and loving parts of your personality, you will not be able to distinguish between frightened and loving parts of other personalities either. A "passion to protect the environment," for example, may come from love or from fear. When I stood in clearcuts that extended as far as I could see and hated the timber industry, my passion came from fear (powerlessness). When I am grateful for Mother Earth, my life, and awed by the exquisitely beautiful and delicate ecology around me, my passion comes from love. Protecting the environment in order to feel worthy or superior is a fear-born passion. Protecting the environment without making others villains because you love Life is a love-born passion. Compassion comes naturally when you can experience all of your passions (frightened parts of your personality and loving parts of your personality) and realize that others have frightened and loving parts of their personalities, too.

- **Experience the Universe as Compassionate and Wise.** If you lived in a white house you would not need to trust that it is white. If friends moved you into a new house while you were on a trip, you would have to trust them that your new house is the color they tell you until you could see it for yourself. The more you trust your friends, the less doubt you would have about the color of your new house, but you could never be certain until you saw it yourself. When you embark on the spiritual path, you trust that the Universe is compassionate and wise because intuition and some of your experiences tell you (or at least you are open to the possibility). As you create authentic power and spiritual partnerships, your experiences show you surprising and beautiful results. Eventually you see opportunities for spiritual growth in each of your experiences, including those that are painful, and in the experiences of others also. Then the compassion and wisdom of the Universe no longer require belief, because you experience them yourself. This is the experience that you were born to live.

The benefits of spiritual partnership are not available to passersby, casual shoppers, or spiritual tourists. They require participation in spiritual partnerships. Spiritual partnerships are arenas for discovering and challenging your fears and exploring and cultivating your love with others. They are joint experiments, bold ventures into the eternally new territory of the eternal present moment. The changes that you make in yourself are permanent. You can ignore what you see and learn, but you cannot unlearn or unsee it. Once you explore frightened and loving parts of your personality, you will recognize them when they become active and the necessity of choosing between them. You may create constructive consequences or destructive consequences, but you will no longer be able to deny that you are responsible for what you create.

The dynamics that produce emptiness and pain—the Universal Laws of Creation, Cause and Effect, and Attraction—also produce joy and meaning depending upon the choices that you make. Spiritual partners experiment with these dynamics and help one another choose wisely.

18
Soul Summary

SPIRITUAL PARTNERSHIPS—BENEFITS

- The benefit of spiritual partnership is authentic power.
- Authentic power is the life that your heart longs to live—fulfilled, grateful, caring, patient, fully present, meaningful, creative, and loving.
- Using spiritual partnerships wisely satisfies the needs of the loving parts of your personality. It creates heaven on Earth, and no matter what happens—no matter what happens—you live in it.

When you realize these things about spiritual partnership, the most important question you can think of, the question that most urgently requires an answer, the question you have been asking all your life becomes, *How* do I create spiritual partnerships? *How* do I become authentically empowered? *How* do I support others in creating authentic power?

Now is always the time to ask and answer that question. Read on.

HOW

19

The Spiritual Partnership Guidelines

The creation of authentic power is a process, not an event. It unfolds moment by moment in response to ever-changing and never-the-same circumstances. Even circumstances that appear to be the same, such as a repetitive experience of overwhelm or an ongoing power struggle, are not really the same. Like a snowflake, each moment is unique, combining different states of consciousness, intentions, and actions. Unlike a snowflake, the complexity of each moment is far more intricate and involved than a geometrical form can be. You are different at each moment, and so are those around you. Authentic power is created (or not) in this kaleidoscopically changing context, each turn of the kaleidoscope bringing new opportunities and challenges.

An argument, for example, can turn quickly into a friendly resolution, and a friendly exchange can turn as quickly into a misunderstanding. Frightened or loving parts of your personality are activated and contribute their thoughts, intentions, words, and actions each moment. The same dynamic occurs in those with whom you interact. No formula or set of rules can guide you through the depth and richness of a moment, much less a life of moments as they present themselves. You cannot predetermine your responses, because you do not know what the next moment will bring. You do not even know whether or not you will be in the Earth school the next moment, much less what others will do.

The same type of calculations that can predict where and when a rocket that is launched from the Earth will arrive on

Mars cannot predict what you or others will choose in the next moment. Others are no more constrained in their choices than you are in yours. Your body is subject to physical regularities (for example, it accelerates according to the law of gravity when you jump from a diving platform), but your will has no constraints. You can intend whatever you choose. Throughout the constantly changing richness of the present moment your capacity to choose remains constant. Philosophy, theology, psychology, and physiology address our ability to respond to change, but they are adventures into thought that, like all such excursions, are limited by the intellect.

Multisensory individuals are not limited by the intellect. Their adventures go far beyond it. The intellect is an employee of multisensory individuals, not the employer. They use the intellect to help them understand authentic power and the tools that are necessary to create it, but applying those tools takes them into domains of experience that the intellect cannot anticipate or grasp. As you become multisensory you begin to use your intellect instead of allowing your intellect to use you. Imagine a child learning to garden who realizes for the first time that she can use her toy shovel to plant flowers instead of vegetables. A big change has occurred. The tool no longer determines how she will use it. She decides how she will use the tool.

An individual who understands authentic power for the first time—what it is, how it is created, and why it is necessary—is like a gardener arriving for the first time at a perfect plot with the intention to grow the best garden possible. Without her intention the plot will not change and a garden will not appear. Your perfect plot is your life. Without your intention to challenge and heal the frightened parts of your personality you will remain angry, jealous, resentful, needing to please, needing to dominate, judging others, judging yourself, and in countless other painful ways continue to mask the pain of powerlessness. Obsessive thoughts (such as "I am so stupid," "I am worthless," "I am to blame," and "I am not loved"), compulsive needs (such as workaholism, perfectionism, and savior searching), and addictive behaviors (such as smoking, drinking, overeating, sex, watching pornography, and gambling) will continue to appear. These are the weeds that are growing in your plot when you discover it. Day by day, month by month, they prevent the growth of the plants that you want to cultivate, such as gratitude, patience, appreciation, and contentment.

Spiritual partners are gardeners on adjoining plots. They share knowledge, experience, and skills. They share love, trust, and the commitment to create authentic power. Their lives are much more complex than gardens, but they share the fundamental feature of all gardens: Unless the gardener pulls the weeds they will continue to grow, and unless the gardener cultivates the flowers they will not bloom. The tools that are necessary to pull the weeds and cultivate the flowers in your garden are emotional awareness, responsible choice, intuition, and trust in the Universe. The more you use them, the more you create authentic power. When creating authentic power is your highest priority, you use them continually.

Only practice can make a gardener. Commitment to gardening and diligently gardening separate those who read about gardening from those who actually work with the soil and experiment, observe, and marvel as shoots emerge, grow into plants, yield fruit, give seeds, and disappear. The beauty and power of the experience cannot be found in a book. Nonetheless, books can be helpful to novice gardeners and experienced gardeners alike.

Without understanding the purpose of your life (garden) and developing the tools to cultivate it, you will exhaust and frustrate yourself, sometimes doing something well, sometimes not, and other times not knowing. These are experiences of an "unexamined life" (Plato's term). A more modern term would be "unconscious life." A still more accurate term would be "reactive life," a life that is frequently controlled by frightened parts of your personality. The transformation of an unexamined, unconscious, reactive life into an aware, deliberate, and joyful life is the creation of authentic power.

Spiritual partners learn how to distinguish between love and fear, choose responsibly, consult intuition, and cocreate with the living Universe. Their experiences together propel them into new domains, and they explore those domains together. The Spiritual Partnership Guidelines help them. Spiritual partners use the Spiritual Partnership Guidelines continually. They are easy to understand, but only applying them can transform the experiences of a victim into those of a creator, and the frustrating and painful pursuit of external power into the gratifying and fulfilling creation of authentic power.

Just as gardening is the only way to become a gardener, the only way to create spiritual partnerships is to create authentic power. The Spiritual Partnership Guidelines show you the most effective, easy-to-use ways to create authentic power in any circumstance at any time. The more you refer to them, the more you will use them, and the more you use them, the more a part of your consciousness they will become. No matter what challenges arise, depression descends, or rage ignites within you—or impatience, superiority, inferiority, need to please, jealousy, obsession, compulsion, addiction, or brutality you encounter from others—the Spiritual Partnership Guidelines will show you how to use it to create authentic power. When you use the Spiritual Partnership Guidelines no wind can blow that does not fill your sails.

The Spiritual Partnership Guidelines are also Authentic Power Guidelines. When you use them you create authentic power no matter what others are doing. Whether you consider them guidelines for creating spiritual partnerships or guidelines for creating authentic power, they are your most effective resource outside of your emotions and intuition. They will remind you to experience your emotions and consult intuition, and help you do it. Their sole and soul purpose is to assist you in creating authentic power and spiritual partnerships.

The Spiritual Partnership Guidelines do not instruct, direct, or command. They are not moral imperatives, philosophical conclusions, or theological instructions. Like findings shared in a journal for the validation or disproof of fellow scientists, the Spiritual Partnership Guidelines are hypotheses that scientists of the soul validate or disprove for themselves in the intimacy of their own experiences. They always point the scientist toward her healthiest options, help her find her bearings when she is lost, and help her at all times to create authentic power.

The Spiritual Partnership Guidelines will continue to evolve as we create authentic power and spiritual partnerships and share our discoveries with one another. Whatever new guidelines emerge, they will support you rather than burden you, open you to curiosity and creativity rather than confine you to dogma, illuminate your potential rather than hide it, contrast your love with your fear, your joy with your happiness, and your fulfillment with your accomplishments to bring your attention again and again to the power of your choices.

In whatever form, the Spiritual Partnership Guidelines (Authentic Power Guidelines) will always direct your attention to your emotions, the force field of your soul; assist you in developing awareness of your emotions; and support you in using your emotions—specifically, your awareness of physical sensations in certain areas of your body such as your chest, solar plexus, and throat—to create authentic power. They will illuminate the fundamental role of your choices and the nature and power of your intentions, and support you in making choices that create consequences for which you are willing to assume responsibility. They will assist you in making intuition instead of intellect your principle decision-making faculty, and support you in using intuition. They will bring the intentions of your soul—harmony, cooperation, sharing, and reverence for Life—to the foreground of your experiences and endeavors, and they will help you use them to measure the spiritual effectiveness of your potential thoughts, words, and actions. As multisensory perception replaces five-sensory perception and millions of us move into an expanded awareness of ourselves and our world, the Spiritual Partnership Guidelines will become more and more valuable to more and more people.

Only spiritual partnerships enhance, deepen, and make more accessible the ongoing opportunities that the Earth school continually provides you to experience and heal frightened parts of your personality and to experience and cultivate loving parts of your personality. They are designed to help you do the following, among other things:

- Use your relationships to create authentic power.
- Communicate consciously and constructively.
- Become courageous in a healthy way.
- Have compassion for yourself and others.
- Act with integrity.
- Support others when they have frightened parts of their personalities active by encouraging them, without attachment, to challenge the frightened parts of their personalities; and by creating authentic power yourself whether or not others decide to challenge the frightened parts of their personalities.
- Support others when they have loving parts of their personalities active by encouraging them, without attachment, to cultivate the loving parts of their personalities; and by creating authentic power yourself whether or not others decide to cultivate the loving parts of their personalities.

The Spiritual Partnership Guidelines do not require belief. They lead to trust in the Universe through your experiences. Multisensory perception allows you to see everyday experiences from the perspective of the soul instead of the perspective of the personality, and makes visible the wisdom and compassion within each experience, at each moment, for each individual. This is not a mystical perception. It is a multisensory perception that emerges more and more clearly as love and trust replace fear and doubt and the constructive consequences of creating authentic power and spiritual partnerships become undeniable.

Multisensory perception is a ready-to-use gift from the Universe. You need only unwrap it and use it. Authentic power is a potential that comes with multisensory perception. It needs to be created, and you can create it only in yourself. The Spiritual Partnership Guidelines are a special-edition travelers' guide for voyagers (like us) who are traversing the terrain of the Earth school recently illuminated by multisensory perception, temporarily participating in experiences of space, time, matter, and duality as we learn through our choices how to align our personalities with our souls and give the gifts that our souls desire to give. They take us through commitment, courage, compassion, and conscious communications and actions step-by-step, pointing out the power, beauty, and necessity of each as we journey from unempowered to empowered—from fear to Love, emptiness to meaning, and pain to joy.

20

Commitment

COMMITMENT—MAKING MY SPIRITUAL GROWTH (CREATING AUTHENTIC POWER) MY HIGHEST PRIORITY

Of all the things I love about Hawaiian culture, I love Aloha best. It is probably the best-known part of Hawaiian culture even though it is difficult to explain. It is not difficult to experience. When an individual has Aloha he radiates joy, appreciation, welcome, and Love. Aloha is open, accepting, and powerful. It nurtures Life and is nurtured by Life. Individuals with Aloha are lighthearted. I have seen Aloha in my Sioux uncle who adopted me and in Tibetan monks. It is unmistakable. I feel appreciated, listened to, and joyfully received. I also feel safe to ask substantive questions and explore meaningful topics. The more I experience Aloha, the more I welcome others into my life. I often marvel that some Hawaiians keep Aloha alive within themselves when so much has been taken from the Hawaiian people.

I marvel at our Native relatives for the same reason. How can some of them keep ancient traditions of healing, wisdom, and compassion, even for the descendants of those who betrayed, abused, and killed their ancestors? Where does their strength come from?

I marvel at African Americans who choose love instead of anger, constructive contribution to the present instead of revenge for the past, for the same reasons. Martin Luther King Jr. and Malcolm X are among my heroes. When I learned that Martin was once so incapacitated by depression that he could not dress himself, my admiration for him knew no bounds. What kept him steadfast on his loving course? What kept Gandhi centered in prison, during beatings, and while religious war swirled around him? What allowed Viktor Frankl, in a Nazi death camp, to see in a moment that changed his life that the Nazis could not take his ability to love from him?

Individuals young and old, female and male, from every culture and race who use their courage to experience the depth of their fears and act on their love inspire me. Some are widely known and others are unknown except to those whose lives they bless. All share the commitment to act in love instead of fear. As we become multisensory we begin to share the same heroes, or at least admire the same commitment to love whenever we see it.

Everyone is committed to something. If you are not sure what your commitments are (and even if you think you know), look around and you will see them reflected to you. When I was a soldier I strove for praise, admiration, and sex. I did not think in terms of commitments, but if I could have seen myself from an impersonal perspective I could have recognized how strong were my commitments to sex and admiration. These goals were so constant and familiar that I did not recognize them as commitments or realize that other commitments were possible. Nonetheless, that did not prevent them from shaping my experiences and creating consequences as effectively as any consciously considered, consciously selected, and consciously held commitment.

Most individuals are committed to creating external power even if they think they are committed to healthy goals such as raising a family or protecting the environment. They have not yet discovered their deepest intentions. Others know that they are committed to creating external power. In both cases (aware of commitment to external power and not aware of commitment to external power), the pursuit of external power is a destructive dead end.

When I wrote *The Dancing Wu Li Masters* I was engaged, excited, and joyful. I knew that I was creating for others, especially those who would come after me with an interest in quantum physics. These experiences were impossible not to notice because they were so new and different for me. Instead of being judgmental and jealous, I admired and appreciated the founders of the quantum theory, some of them as young at the time they created it as I was when I wrote about them. Instead of worrying about paying my rent, I awoke each morning eager to write. If I could have seen myself from an impersonal perspective, I would have seen my commitment to giving others an empowering gift that was joyful for me to create.

If you could see yourself from an impersonal perspective, you would be able to see at once whether your commitment is to love or fear. If you are frequently angry, resentful, or jealous; shout or withdraw emotionally; think judgmental thoughts or search for a savior; indulge in workaholism or perfectionism; are irresistibly attracted to alcohol, sex, drugs, or gambling; or have violent or sexual fantasies and you do not challenge the power of these experiences over you, you are committed to fear. Even if you think you are committed to your religion, nation, culture, ideals (such as harmony, cooperation, sharing, and reverence for Life) or goals (such as protecting the environment or ending a war), you are committed to fear.

Love and fear are the two great commitments of the human experience. They are mutually exclusive. Frightened and loving parts of the personality sometimes become active simultaneously (this is the experience of a splintered personality, for example, I love my brother but I don't like him), but your commitment determines which one you act on. If you are committed to fear, you react. If you are committed to love, you respond (choose responsibly). If you are committed to love and you react instead of respond, you will return to the experience in your mind, learn from it, and use what you learned to help you respond with love next time.

Every frightened part of the personality is committed to fear (pursuing external power), every loving part is committed to love (creating authentic power), and you must choose between them. What others choose is beside the point. Your choice is the point. Commitment to fear raises and crushes hopes, exhilarates and disappoints, succeeds and fails. Commitment to love fulfills, uplifts, validates, and blesses. Your commitment guides your choices, and your choices create your experiences.

Love and fear are the poles of the human experience. Together they encompass every possible human action. They are the signature experiences of the Earth school, requiring each individual to choose between them at each moment. Only the commitment to love allows you to choose love when the magnetic attraction of fear is great—for example, when the need for a drink is overwhelming, or anger erupts uncontrollably in you, or you feel that you must win a power struggle. Only the commitment to fear can prevent love from filling your life and bringing you together with others who are committed to love.

Without the commitment to love you cannot choose love when a frightened part of your personality is active. You will shout, withdraw, exploit emotionally, sexually, or psychologically, drink, overeat, smoke, or take a drug instead. In numerous familiar ways you will mask the pain of powerlessness with an obsessive thought, compulsive action, or addictive behavior. Each time, you anesthetize yourself temporarily, but the anesthetic will wear off. When you commit to love, the Universe assists you. Support for your healthiest choice is always at hand. Even if the part of your personality that wants health is a very small part, it is the part that the Universe backs. That is why commitment to love always transforms, heals, and opens new avenues of creativity.

There are degrees of commitment. Sometimes a commitment

to love is immediate, deep, and clear. Even in the midst of painful emotions the strength of her commitment allows an individual to regain her balance and perspective. A Native American friend, for example, told me how he stopped drinking many years before. "I was walking home drunk one night when I fell down and I couldn't get up," he said. "I was lying facedown in the dirt when I vomited, but I couldn't move. I wanted to get up, but no one was there to help me. I was disgusted with myself. After a while I said to myself, 'This will never happen again.' " It didn't. Now his nonprofit organization teaches Native wisdom to businesses and government agencies.

Other individuals are curious. Their commitment to love is not deep, but it is sufficient to bring them to the idea of authentic power. Sometimes they hear about authentic power on a television show, visit our website, or read a book like this one. The commitment to creating authentic power, or even to experimenting with it, puts an individual on the spiritual path or takes her further along it.

Each time you experience for yourself that you do not need to be controlled by your anger, jealousy, resentment, or craving for food, sex, alcohol, or gambling, you begin to experience some mastery in your life that was not there before. The relationship between your choices and your experiences becomes undeniable and then liberating. Even a small taste of mastery is enough to remind you when you are upset, enraged, or despairing that you do not need to remain in the control of your fears. You do not need to remain thirsty after you have found the well. Each time you challenge a frightened part of your personality you drink from the well again, and the grip of the frightened part of your personality loosens. Eventually it disappears. A flame is ignited and the more brightly it burns in you, the more it illuminates your personality and the opportunities that frightened and loving parts of your personality offer you to grow spiritually.

The more you drink from the well, the less you need a commitment to return. Do you need a commitment to drink when you are thirsty, eat when you are hungry, or rest when you are tired? Your wholeness calls to you, attracting your attention regardless of which frightened parts of your personality are active—which painful sensations are flaring, pounding, burning, stabbing, or aching in your body; which depressing, judgmental, or violent thoughts they are thinking; or what hopelessness or helplessness they are experiencing. A new and healthy potential emerges, only one choice away. The more you choose it, the more you bring it into your life.

Commitment to love—to spiritual growth, to creating authentic power—is a down-in-the-soil, everyday application of your will to use each of your experiences to create constructive instead of destructive consequences, harmony instead of discord, to share instead of hoard, cooperate instead of compete, and revere Life instead of exploit Life. It is the determination to act from the healthiest parts of your personality, create more joy and less pain, more meaning and less emptiness, and more love and less fear in your life no matter what. The commitment to love makes Aloha possible. Nothing else can. It keeps Native traditions alive. Nothing else can. It enables slaves and descendants of slaves to love instead of hate. Nothing else can. It empowered Viktor Frankl, Martin Luther King Jr., Gandhi, and Malcolm X to open their hearts. Nothing else could. It enables you to finally, at last, challenge and heal the frightened parts of your personality and cultivate the loving parts.

Nothing else can.

21

Commitment Guidelines

In this chapter are a few ways of looking at the Spiritual Partnership Guidelines, beginning with the commitment guidelines. There are many more, and as you practice with the Spiritual Partnership Guidelines you will discover your own ways. Once you understand something in its simplicity you can explain it in any vocabulary, in any culture, and to any age group. Creating authentic power is simple. Learn to distinguish fear from love, and choose love. Open to your multisensory perception. Apply your courage, and make different choices. Now is the time to create authentic power and spiritual partnerships—now while the human experience is changing; now while old ways of interacting have become toxic and new healthy ways are appearing; now while you have the insight, or impulse, or vision to change your life into what it can be without fear.

• **FOCUS ON WHAT I CAN LEARN ABOUT MYSELF all the time, especially from my reactions (such as anger, fear, jealousy, resentment, and impatience), instead of judging or blaming others or myself.**

This is the heart of spiritual growth, the heart of creating authentic power, and the heart of cocreating with the Universe: Change yourself. Allow yourself to be flexible and limber instead of rigid and righteous. Assume that your emotional distress—all of it—has to do with you and you alone. What others do that you find stressful may or may not be experienced as stressful by all. If others had the power to cause you emotional pain, you would spend your entire life—day after day—attempting to manipulate

or control them in order to avoid it. You would be ever obser-
vant, always on alert for possible pain, and you would develop
sensitivities to your vulnerabilities and ways to protect yourself
from exposing them. You would learn to please, impress, intimi-
date, dominate, or terrify others in order to feel safe and valuable. This is the pursuit of external power. Most people pursue
external power continually. Every individual and circumstance
is assessed for its capability to make you feel safe and valuable or
to invalidate your values, belittle your abilities, and deflate your
sense of well-being. You open yourself only when you do not feel
threatened, and then only as necessary. What passes for relaxation occurs only in the company of those who think, look, act,
and believe like you—and thoughts, appearances, actions, and
beliefs can change quickly.

You fear displeasing even those who love you, such as parents
and grandparents or those who have taken their places in your
life, and especially those you most need (such as parents and
grandparents or those who have taken their places). You fear that
authorities will impose their will upon yours, attempt to please
those who can give you what you feel you need, and fear those
who want what you have. The more you acquire, the more you fear
losing it. Everyone becomes suspect. The angrier you become, the
angrier the people around you become. The more impatient you
become, the more people around you become impatient.

The world becomes a threatening place with few, if any,
moments of respite. You cannot change yourself except to adapt to
new circumstances, new threats, and new dangers to your sense
of purpose and value. The more frightened you become the more
defensive you become, and the less you are able to see others and
your circumstances clearly, if at all. You surround yourself with
those who appear least threatening and defend yourself against
those who appear most threatening. These are the experiences
of an unexamined life (philosophical term), an unconscious life
(psychological term), an empty life (existential term), a pain-

ful life (street term), and frightened parts of your personality (vocabulary of authentic power).

While you focus on people and external circumstances, you look away from the causes of all these painful experiences—the frightened parts of your personality that you were born to discover (experience) and heal (by not acting on them)—and from the causes of all your fulfilling and joyful experiences—the loving parts of your personality that you were born to discover (experience) and strengthen (by acting on them). Creating authentic power is radically different in every way from pursuing external power. Instead of attempting to change others in order to feel safe and valuable, you find the interior sources of your self-disgust, self-dislike, and self-hatred and heal them; and you find the interior sources of your gratitude, patience, and appreciation and cultivate them. Your endeavors to change the world become more focused because you know exactly how to change it most effectively and permanently: Change in yourself what you want to change in the world. If you want to see less jealousy in the world, become less jealous. If you want to see less rage in the world, become less angry. If you want to see more love in the world, become more loving. This is an ambitious program and the only one that now offers you the potential of meaning, fulfillment, and joy.

• **PAY ATTENTION TO MY EMOTIONS by feeling the physical sensations in my energy centers (such as my chest, solar plexus, and throat areas).**

Using your body to grow spiritually grounds you in the reality of your emotions. It brings you into the present moment. Nothing is more effective in taking you out of your fantasies, imaginings, and daydreams. In fact, these are ways of avoiding your emotions. In predigital days when newspapers were the primary source of news, newsboys shouted headlines from their street stands to attract buyers: "New Front Opens in France!" "Battle of Britain Intensifies!" "Stock Market Climbs!" Your emotions are like the newsboys, shouting important news to attract your attention. Ignoring them is like disregarding a messenger who has important information. Emotional headlines are even clearer. "Pain in Right Center of Chest!" "Churning in Stomach!" "Relaxation in Throat!" "Openness in Chest!" They never stop. When you tune in to them you receive a constant update on your emotional status. The headlines (emotions) continue whether or not you are aware of them. If you are not, you cannot benefit from them.

The headlines do not shout "Jealousy," "Rage," "Appreciation," "Gratitude," etc. These are labels, not emotions. The headlines skip the labels and go directly to the emotional experience. That is what you get when you pay attention to them—direct, unfiltered, unlabeled experiences of emotions. Nothing stands between you and them. You feel them in your body. Distinct and defined sensations come and go continually, each combining into headlines that frequently change. The news is always current.

If you can't read, newspapers can't help you. If you can, they provide you information for your benefit. If you don't understand your painful emotions (and do your best to avoid them, for example, by judging, gambling, drinking, having sex, etc.), or you do not understand your blissful, pleasing emotions (and don't explore them, for example, by assuming that they are caused by others or by circumstances), you can't benefit from your emotions any more than someone who is illiterate can benefit from newspapers. If you can, you can use what your emotions show you to change your life for the better. When the sensations that you feel near an energy center (such as your throat, chest, or solar plexus) are uncomfortable or painful, a frightened part of your personality is active regardless of what you are thinking, imagining, or doing. When they are pleasing, a loving part is active regardless of what you are thinking, imagining, or doing. This is the priceless information. Your body will not lie to you.

When you know that a frightened part of your personality is active, you can act accordingly—specifically, not do what it wants (for example, not shout, criticize, withdraw, etc.). Frightened parts of your personality always create painful consequences (such as pushing people away, isolation, loneliness, lack of intimacy, and so on). If you do not know when they are active, they will create these consequences for you. If you recognize when a frightened part of your personality is active and you do not act as it desires, you spare yourself these painful experiences (karma) and at the same time weaken the frightened part of your personality that would create more of them. If you recognize when a loving part of your personality is active and you act on it, you assure yourself fulfilling and blissful experiences in the future (karma) and at the same time strengthen the loving part of your personality that will create more of them. This is spiritual growth.

Be patient. Sometimes you will feel painful sensations near some energy centers and pleasing sensations near others. The first are processing the energy flowing through them in fear and doubt, and the second are processing it in love and trust. This is an experience of a splintered personality (loving and frightened parts of your personality are active at the same time). The complexity of your emotional experiences reflects the complexity of your life.

• **PAY ATTENTION TO MY THOUGHTS (such as judging, analyzing, comparing, daydreaming, planning my reply, etc., or thoughts of gratitude, appreciation, contentment, openness to Life, etc.).**

Sometimes it takes practice to develop emotional awareness. It is a developmental process, like learning to read. Some people are more skilled at it than others. (Don't be fooled: someone who throws her emotions around, for example, becomes hysterical, weepy, and angry easily, is emotionally indulgent, not emotionally aware. This won't help her to grow spiritually, and it pushes people away.) If you cannot feel your emotions as physical sensations in your body, keep trying. They are there, and you will find them. (When you are upset, they will find you.) In the meanwhile, your thoughts will give you the same information. If you are thinking judgmental, critical, angry, violent, sexually exploiting, or grieving thoughts, a frightened part of your personality is active. Loving parts of your personality think thoughts of gratitude, appreciation, patience, contentment, etc. When you are thinking thoughts like these, a loving part of your personality is active. That is a part of your personality that you were born to cultivate, nurture, and bring to the foreground of your awareness and life.

Even if you feel your emotions as sensations near your energy centers, you can still monitor your thoughts at the same time. You will always see a correlation between them and your emotions. Painful sensations occur at the same time as thoughts that are critical, angry, frightened, judgmental, etc. Pleasing sensations occur at the same time as thoughts that are forgiving, caring, patient, grateful, and so on. Use this information the same way. Challenge the frightened parts of your personality when they are active (don't act on them), and cultivate the loving parts when they are active (act on them). When you do this, the frightened parts of your personality begin to lose their influence over you, and the loving parts become more noticeable and attractive to you.

• **PAY ATTENTION TO MY INTENTION (such as blaming, judging, needing to be right, seeking admiration, escaping into thoughts (intellectualizing), trying to convince, etc., or cooperating, sharing, creating harmony, and revering Life).**

Noticing your intention is something like noticing your future. Your intentions create your experiences. When you know what you intend, you know what you are creating, and the experiences that you create will not surprise you when you encounter them. Intentions that you do not know about (your unconscious intentions) create as powerfully as those that you know about, but since you do not know about them, you are unaware of what you are creating. The experiences that unconscious intentions create always surprise you when they come, and they are never pleasant. Someone who caretakes others in order to feel worthy and valuable, for example, eventually becomes frustrated and then angry when her efforts are unappreciated. "What is wrong with these people!" she exclaims. "I care for them. I am patient with them. I am there for them. And they do not appreciate me!" Her care is sticky. It comes with hidden agendas, for example, the need to be appreciated. People feel her need, and they do not want to pay the price for her "care." She cares for herself, not them. If she were aware of her intention she could change it, and the consequences that it creates would change also.

During the Cold War a woman built an underground shelter on her property. She thought that her intention was to care for others. "I have stored enough food in my shelter to feed one hundred people for a year," she proclaimed. Actually, she had stored enough food to feed herself for one hundred years. She was not aware of her real intention, but that was the intention that created consequences for her. It did not attract people who care about her. It attracted people who tell themselves that they care about others but actually care about themselves.

Intention is the key to the kingdom, any kingdom (or queendom). That is why it is so important to examine carefully the key you are selecting. Some kingdoms are not inviting (such as the kingdoms of greed, fear, exploitation, competition, and discord), and some are (such as the kingdoms of gratitude, contentment, appreciation, and joy). When you choose the key, it opens its kingdom. If you do not know what kingdom your key will open, you will after you choose it. Why not examine the keys that you are considering closely before you choose one? No one likes to live in a violent, brutal, and avaricious kingdom, but many people do. They see themselves as kind or patient, except when they become angry, enraged, judgmental, etc. (frightened parts of their personalities become active). These are especially good times to examine the keys you are choosing.

Excavate as deeply as you can to find your intention before you act and the consequences that it creates will not surprise you. If they do, dig deeper before you act the next time.

22

Courage

COURAGE—STRETCHING MYSELF BEYOND THE LIMITED PERSPECTIVES OF THE FRIGHTENED PARTS OF MY PERSONALITY

Multisensory individuals use courage in a way that five-sensory individuals do not consider. When I was in the army, for example, courage meant to me, among other things, parachuting with equipment at night. Every parachute jump requires a main parachute, which is strapped to the back of the jumper, and a small reserve chute strapped to the front. Equipment jumps require, in addition, a heavy equipment bag which is attached below the reserve chute. After the main chute deploys, the jumper releases the bag and it falls to the end of a long elastic cord where it hangs, allowing it to hit the ground first a safe distance away from the jumper. When the jumper is on the ground he follows the cord to the bag and retrieves the content. Last comes the rifle, strapped to the side of the jumper, muzzle up. This was one of the most worrisome parts of each jump for me. A good parachute landing fall requires a kind of tumbling roll, which I never learned how to do with a rifle strapped to me like a torso-length splint.

Since all of this happens in the dark, the unnaturalness of jumping out of an airplane, trying to do it well, hoping the canopy deploys, hoping that if it doesn't the reserve chute deploys, remembering to release the equipment bag, the deafening noise of the aircraft and sudden quietness of falling through the air, trying to reach the drop zone, hoping the wind does not pick up, seeing the ground rush toward me out of the darkness, fearing a landing on rocks or being dragged or both, and trying to do a parachute landing fall in a splint combined to make the experience totally terrifying for me, yet I did it again and again.

Even before that, after quitting college and traveling to Europe, I sat on a street bench in Stockholm with my guitar, summoning my courage to sing in public for money. I determined to stay there until I stood up and played, no matter how long it took. I sat there for several hours before I was finally able. I was very frightened but I did it anyway, partly because I was hungry and partly because I would not let my fear prevent me from doing what I wanted to do.

These are examples of the old courage, the courage to do what is necessary in order to feel accepted, valuable, and safe. Children (and adults) taunt one another to demonstrate the old courage. "Are you a baby?" has been enough to launch countless foolish acts, such as jumping from a cliff into a river without knowing the depth of the water or "playing chicken" with oncoming cars. I used the old courage to lead Top Secret missions into Laos and to run rapids on the Colorado River in a kayak instead of in the oar boats that most of our party used. Doing these things made me feel special. I didn't see at the time that they covered my pain of powerlessness.

Spiritual growth requires the courage to use your will to heal your own fears instead of trying to change everyone else. This is not the recklessness of a daredevil who breaks thirty bones and survives (as a friend did in a climbing accident) or parachuting with combat equipment (as I did). It is the courage to keep the commitment to yourself to experience and heal all of the frightened parts of your personality instead of indulge them or run from them.

Whether or not the frightened parts of your personality heal depends upon your intention. For example, climbing a mountain requires courage, but if your reason for climbing it is recognition or self-validation, the climb itself is an act of fear. This is an example of the old courage. The climb does not challenge your pain of powerlessness but actually reinforces it. I have a friend who is proud of his dramatic rags-to-riches story, a truly remarkable journey from poverty to superwealth, but the fuel for his ascent into material wealth was the need to prove to himself that he has value, that he has his place in the world, and that he is worth knowing and being with. Creating authentic power requires stretching yourself instead of remaining in the fortress of familiar fears.

For example, suppose you have something that you know you need to say and you don't say it because you are intimidated or feel unworthy to speak. That is a way of keeping yourself separate from the intimacy that is possible when you share, even when you are having an emotional reaction such as anger, fear, jealousy, need to please, need to withdraw, and so on. Speaking with the intention of reducing the distance that you feel from an individual instead of making him wrong requires courage. Withdrawing, creating an internal distance between you, silently judging, and remaining in a power struggle do not.

On the other hand, if you usually speak frequently or continually and you feel the urge to speak yet again, speaking does not require courage. In this case, the irresistible urge to intrude your perception, impose yourself, explain yourself, or set the record straight masks the pain of powerlessness. Challenging that urge by not speaking and instead experiencing the sensations in your body, which are uncomfortable, requires courage. The dynamic is the same in each instance—challenging what you compulsively feel you must do in the moment, whether it is to speak or remain silent, brings to the surface of your awareness uncomfortable sensations in your body that lie beneath the need. These are direct experiences of frightened parts of your personality. Doing what you have always done to mask these sensations, to make yourself comfortable again, does not require courage. In fact, that is spiritual cowardice.

When I met Linda I was grieving the dissolution of my engagement. My former fiancée and I had separated five years earlier, but I still clung to the future we had envisioned. At the same time, my relationship with Linda was like none I had experienced—not sexual or romantic but engaging and meaningful, even when I did not enjoy being with her. I decided to explore the possibility of reconnecting with my ex-fiancée one last time before I opened to the new experiences I was having with Linda, so I called her. She was not interested. That very evening during a candlelight dinner in my cabin Linda asked me if I had called my ex-fiancée to ask about getting together again. No one except my ex-fiancée knew about our call. I was (very) surprised and suddenly in a circumstance I had not experienced before. If I lied to Linda I would destroy the very thing that made our relationship special. If I told her the truth, I risked losing it.

She waited patiently for my answer. At last I told her about my call and what my ex-fiancée and I discussed. I shared the pain I had felt for five long years and my aching for the dreams we had shared. I held my breath and waited for Linda to stand, leave the table, and leave my life, but she remained sitting, still looking at me. At last she said, "I am glad you told me. Now I can love her, too."

Suddenly I was in a new realm. I had told the truth and the worst had not happened, although I was prepared for it. The best had happened instead. Linda remained. I felt deeper relief than I could have imagined. Not only did Linda stay in my life, but our relationship deepened and became stronger. I had challenged my fear for new and different reasons than I had in the past. I challenged it for health, for wholeness, for love. Attempting to manipulate Linda, especially Linda, was not acceptable to me.

When I answered Linda truthfully, I opened a door to experiences that I did not know existed. I felt at home in the Universe, at ease, in awe of the miracle of Life, and grateful for it. In the past I had used my courage in the service of gaining admiration, success, recognition, a Green Beret, and sex. This time I used it in the service of my integrity. I wanted to build my relationship with Linda, if I was going to have one, on a foundation of trust, not on the sand of a falsehood. I feared losing my relationship with her, but sacrificing my integrity to keep it was not an option, because the relationship that I wanted required integrity. This is an example of the new courage.*

I didn't realize at the time that I had discovered the difference between using courage to create external power and using it to create authentic power, between the old courage and the new courage. In the military my need to feel valuable was so deep and the pain of powerlessness so intense that I forced myself to face death if necessary to mask it. My need to build a healthy relationship with Linda was another story. I was not attempting to feel better about myself by impressing her or winning her affection. My goal was to explore the depths of intimacy and new realms of health and cocreativity with her—in short, to cooperate with her, share with her, create harmony with her, and revere her.

The new courage enables spiritual growth. The old courage prevents it. The new courage creates authentic power. The old courage pursues external power. The old courage assuages the pain of powerlessness. The new courage eliminates it. The old courage leads to pride. The new courage leads to fulfillment.

Courage is required when will and fear intersect. Where there is no fear, there is no courage, only will. These are the experiences of the loving parts of your personality. They do not require courage in order to be caring, contented, grateful, appreciative, or to love Life. They are fearless travelers through the Earth school, always expressing the energy of the soul, continually creating

---

* See the "A New Way of Relating" chapter in *Soul Stories* (Gary Zukav, Simon & Schuster, 2000) for another account of this special experience.

with the intentions of the soul. They are fearless not because they are courageous but because they have no fear. They trust the Universe. When you align yourself with one of them instead of with a frightened part of your personality, you align yourself with your soul.

This happens in ways large as well as ways that appear small. For example, when a friend irritates you it takes courage—and a surprising lot of courage—to turn your attention inward, scan your energy centers, experience the physical sensations in your body, and while you are experiencing the pain of this emotion, not act or speak with irritation. Most people do not use their courage this way, and they are controlled by the frightened parts of their personalities. I would not have understood, much less believed, how much more courage it requires to experience the painful sensations of anger, embarrassment, jealousy, or resentment without acting on them than it required for me to do the things that I felt at the time were admirable and dangerous.

For example, I did not have the courage when I enlisted in the infantry to experience how much I feared trying and failing or not living up to my expectations of myself or the expectations that I thought others had of me. Instead I became a paratrooper, then a Green Beret, and then I led Top Secret missions to Top Secret places. These activities allowed me to think that I was courageous. I was, but not enough to experience my emotions when the strongest frightened parts of my personality were active (which they usually were). Fear controlled most of the things that I did, even when I felt courageous.

Macho means "too frightened to consider the possibility of being frightened." I was macho. If someone had suggested to me that I was a Green Beret because I was frightened, I would have exploded in anger (fear) and resentment (fear). I was controlled by external circumstances. Some external circumstances made me feel better (such as when I was admired or successful at a sexual seduction), and some were intensely painful (such as when

I felt that I appeared inadequate or ridiculed). I did not have the courage to turn my attention inward and respond instead of react when a frightened part of my personality was active. I did not have the courage to ask myself, "Why is *that* upsetting me?" In short, I had the old courage but not the new courage.

The new courage is as important for multisensory humans evolving through spiritual growth as the old courage was for five-sensory humans who evolved through survival, but they have different purposes. Five-sensory humans use the old courage to overcome fear in order to explore external circumstances and manipulate or control them. Multisensory humans use the new courage to overcome fear in order to explore internal circumstances and align their personalities with their souls.

23

Courage Guidelines

Five-sensory individuals admire the courage to keep going when they want to give up, the odds are impossible, everything is against them, or everything is falling apart. This is the old courage. Wanting to quit, having no strength to continue, and feeling despair are experiences of frightened parts of the personality. Multisensory humans admire the courage to heal the frightened parts of the personality and cultivate the loving parts. This is the new courage.

Attempting to change a frightened part of your personality into a loving part is like trying to change a tree into a tulip, or a porcupine into a horse. Healing the frightened parts of your personality does not change them. It diminishes their control over you as you repeatedly experience and challenge them until their control over you disappears. That requires the new courage.

- **TAKE RESPONSIBILITY** for my feelings, experiences, and actions (no blaming).

This is the central theme of authentic power. Everything revolves around your taking responsibility for your experiences. When it comes to taking responsibility for what you experience, you either do or you do not. There is no in between.

I tried to hike completely around Mount Shasta above the treeline several times when I lived at its base. Each time, a huge drainage on the north side called Mud Creek stopped me. Despite its unimaginative name, Mud Creek is awesome. An enormous landslide in the mountain's history left a huge cleft that begins at the glaciers near the summit and deepens and widens as it descends thousands of feet. The sides are so steep, the bottom so deep, and the scree so difficult to descend and climb that Mud Creek is impassable for me.

The chasm between taking responsibility for your experiences and not taking responsibility for them is bigger than Mud Creek. It is the gap between five-sensory evolution and multisensory evolution. Five-sensory humans cannot bridge this gap because they see external circumstances as the causes of their emotions. Multisensory humans know better.

Creating authentic power means becoming the authority in your life. Who else knows more about you, feels what you feel, experiences what you experience, and cares for your aspirations more than you? Becoming your own authority means listening to the counsel of others but not necessarily accepting it. For example, if you hear something that resonates with you, who except you is to say, "That is worth remembering" or "That is not worth remembering"? When you have a dream that puzzles, frightens, or enlightens you, who except you can decide to ponder or forget it?

Taking responsibility for your experiences means reminding yourself, whatever is happening, "This is happening for a reason. I may not be able to see the reason now. My intention is to learn all that I can about myself. How can this experience help me heal the fear-based parts of my personality?" Taking responsibility for your experiences is the fundamental challenge to every frightened part of your personality, because none of those parts feel responsible for what they do. The angry parts, for example, are convinced that their anger is caused by others and justified. The jealous parts are convinced that their jealousy is caused by others and justified. The overwhelmed parts are convinced that their overwhelm is caused by circumstances and justified, and so on.

When you take responsibility for all of your experiences, you put yourself in the very powerful position of being able to discover which of your choices created which of your experiences and therefore capable of re-creating them or not. Instead of assuming that others or circumstances create your experiences (this is how a victim sees the world), you assume that your choices create them (this is how a creator sees the world).

Some frightened parts of your personality are so familiar that they seem to be "who you are," and the idea of changing them appears impossible because that would require changing your very essence. This is not accurate. Your essence would surprise you and fill you with joy and wonder without the distorted perceptions of the frightened parts of your personality. Taking responsibility for your experiences enables you to find and heal all of them.

• **PRACTICE INTEGRITY at all times (often requires action, such as speaking when frightened parts of my personality don't want to speak and not speaking when they feel compelled to speak).**

The first and only cruise ship I took stopped in Jamaica. The crowd at the dock was boisterous and, to me, intimidating. Hundreds of people competed loudly to sell paintings, carvings, clothing, and tours. Clothing and art are matters of taste, but hiring a guide warranted careful attention. Officers on the ship warned us about potential unpleasant experiences (such as being robbed), and the message I understood was that different guides take customers to different experiences of Jamaica. Choosing a guide who will take you to the parts of the island that you want to see was the challenge.

Integrity and conscience both present themselves as guides through your life, however, they are distinctly different guides, and they take you to distinctly different places. Conscience takes you where your culture, parents, or peers want you to go. It also discourages you from visiting places that have not been approved by them. When you ignore your conscience you feel guilty and remorseful, as though you have betrayed a trust or disappointed an expectation. In fact, your collective expects certain behaviors from you, but it also does more than that. It imposes nonnegotiable demands.

Conscience tells you when you have ignored a nonnegotiable demand or you are thinking about ignoring one, for example, "Don't lie" (or "Thou shalt not lie," if you speak archaically). Even thinking about ignoring such a demand (command) activates conscience. You feel guilty at the least and terrified, a failure, and condemned to endless pain at worst. These are experiences of frightened parts of your personality. In other words, conscience and fear are the same. Conscience is the painful anticipation of painful punishment. The demands of every collective, no matter how different in content, are all starkly black-and-white, either-or, this or that. Conscience guides you to the painful fear of pain and the painful need to avoid pain. That is its function. It insures that you conform to commands decreed by others or suffer punishments decreed by others.

Psychologists call this "internalizing" an authority. You are not the authority. You are controlled by the authority. Even if the authority is absent, even if it no longer exists (as in the case of a deceased parent), you are controlled by the authority. If you disobey a command and you think that you will never be caught, you still live in the fear (pain) of being caught (and punished). You punish yourself until you are punished by others. The authority takes up residence inside you as your "conscience," and you experience it as fear. Awareness of your conscience and awareness of frightened parts of your personality are identical.

Five-sensory humans feel "out of integrity" when they violate a collective demand. Multisensory humans feel "out of integrity" when they do something that they know is generated by fear instead of love. They feel "in integrity" when they act in love, with compassion and wisdom.

When I decided to quit Harvard I told my roommates, my

friends, and, at last, the dean of students, who asked me, "Have you told your father?" That was the question I least wanted to hear. My father had not gone to college, and his immigrant parents had not gone to high school. Integrity required that I go home to tell him in person that I was dropping out of Harvard. It took all of my courage, but I could not leave without doing it. (I did not know that I would return a year later.)

A friend, Brian Weiss, resigned as chairman of the Department of Psychiatry at Mt. Sinai Hospital to share discoveries of his patients' past-life experiences and teach others how to remember their own. That choice put his medical license, the financial security of his family, and the respect of his peers into potential jeopardy, but his integrity required it. He has since introduced millions of individuals to multisensory perception through books and appearances and validated it in millions more.

You cannot know in advance what integrity will require of you. If you need to speak to keep yourself from feeling uncomfortable, to show people that you are there, or to control the conversation, and you are aware of it, integrity requires not speaking. If speaking in a group intimidates you or you think that what you have to say is not important, and you are aware of it, integrity requires speaking. Each interaction brings its own healing potential. Integrity calls you to that potential. If you ignore it you feel unsettled, on the "wrong track," or wanting to choose again. If you answer the call you feel at ease and content with the path that you have chosen.

Conscience imposes itself upon you. Integrity calls to you. Conscience demands that you listen to frightened parts of your personality and obey them. Integrity requires listening to loving parts of your personality and honoring them. Conscience takes you where others want you to go. Integrity takes you where your soul wants you to go.

• SAY OR DO WHAT IS MOST DIFFICULT (sharing what I notice, if appropriate, when someone speaks or acts from a frightened part of his or her personality; sharing about myself what I am frightened to say and know that I need to say).

Look carefully at your intention before sharing something that is difficult for you to share. Does it come from fear? Are you saying something to judge and blame the other person? Or does it come from love? Do you intend to create a healthier relationship or support another in growing spiritually? Words can do so much healing or create so much damage, especially when you are upset. This guideline does not give you permission to vent, rage, judge, disdain, criticize, or condemn overtly or covertly. In other words, saying what is most difficult does not mean making someone wrong, inferior, or a villain.

Saying what is most difficult for you to say helps you remove the distance you feel from another and speak in real, connected, and appropriate ways. It challenges frightened parts of your personality that think, "If I say this, I will hurt him"; "If I say that, we will not be intimate." The opposite is true. Avoiding what needs to be said destroys intimacy. If you do not have the courage to tell a friend, for example, that his anger frightens you or that her drinking is unacceptable, a distance forms between you and grows.

Frightened parts of your personality will not say what is most difficult because they strive for security and comfort. For example, Linda once asked a circle of students who had studied authentic power with us for several years, "Which of your spiritual partners in this circle do you feel are ready to support new participants in the Authentic Power Program?" Silence filled the room. No one was willing to speak about another in the circle in a way that might jeopardize the relationship between them (this is not spiritual partnership). At last she asked one of the participants directly.

"Everyone here is ready!" he declared quickly. "I would be honored to have anyone here support me." Linda paused for a moment and asked him if he had used the Spiritual Partnership

Guidelines before answering—if he had scanned the physical sensations in his energy centers, noticed his thoughts, and observed his intention for speaking. Then she asked him if he felt that his answer came from a loving part of his personality or a frightened part of his personality. He saw that a frightened part of his personality had declared, "I would be honored to have anyone here support me." He knew that not everyone in the circle was ready to support new participants, and so did his spiritual partners.

Finally, Linda asked him if he could go around the circle, look each person in the eye, and tell each whether or not he felt that he or she was ready to support new participants. This required the courage to take responsibility for his decision, to challenge the frightened part of his personality that did not want to answer the question, to tell each of his spiritual partners one-on-one what he felt. He decided to be in integrity and to say what was most difficult for him, with the intention to support, to those he did not feel were ready as well as to those he did feel were ready.

This decision made a big difference to everyone in the circle. It transformed what could have been a superficial exercise in pleasing and lack of integrity (indulging a frightened part of his personality) into a real-time supportive experience for all. He modeled spiritual partnership and the courage and integrity that it requires. Then each spiritual partner in the circle answered the same question, addressing one another, one at a time. You create authentic power when you say what is most difficult with the intention to challenge and heal a frightened part of your personality. You also create authentic power when you care enough about another to share what you fear might damage your relationship. You create it when you care enough to consider the most appropriate ways to express yourself before you speak.

Saying and doing what is most difficult is not an occasional necessity for spiritual partners. It is an ongoing commitment.

24

Soul Summary

SPIRITUAL PARTNERSHIPS— FROM COURAGE TO COMPASSION

Moving from the old courage—the courage to manipulate and control circumstances and people in order to feel secure and valuable—to compassion (the next section of the Spiritual Partnership Guidelines) is difficult or impossible. Moving from the new courage to compassion—the courage to experience all the parts of your personality, challenge the frightened parts, and cultivate the loving parts—is a natural step.

How can intentionally decreasing fear in your life and intentionally increasing love in your life not lead you directly into compassion?

25

Compassion

COMPASSION—SEEING MYSELF AND OTHERS AS SOULS WHO SOMETIMES HAVE FRIGHTENED PARTS OF THEIR PERSONALITIES ACTIVE

Multisensory perception unveils many experiences that five-sensory humans consider compassion—from warm feelings about cute puppies and kittens, to giving money to homeless people, to funding charitable activities—and reveals them to be something very different from compassion. Compassion is caring about others without second agendas. Every frightened part of your personality pursues external power, and sometimes that agenda is hidden, for example, in a smile that is intended to disarm a client or seduce a potential sexual partner. A smile that comes from a loving part of your personality nurtures, expresses joy, and brings you closer to others.

If you do not know when frightened parts of your personality are active and when loving parts of your personality are active, you cannot distinguish between compassion and fear that masquerades as compassion. Creating authentic power requires this ability. Illuminating all the rooms of your mansion—discovering all of the frightened and loving parts of your personality—makes the differences between fear that appears to be compassion and true compassion visible. When you embark on the spiritual path you will be surprised to discover how much you thought was compassion in yourself and others is not, and how different compassion is from what you might have thought it to be.

Giving money to a homeless person who drinks, for example, is no more compassionate than buying drinks for a wealthy alcoholic. Which parts of your personality see such a gift as compassionate? (Hint: frightened parts.) Which see it as destructive? (Hint: loving parts.) The parts of your personality that fear being moneyless and homeless see any gift to a moneyless and homeless person as compassionate. Homeless people activate these parts of your personality, and these parts give them money to mask the pain of powerlessness. They do not care about the homeless person. The homeless person is an object to these parts of your personality, and a frightening object. When they give the object money, they see themselves for a moment as they would like to see themselves and be seen—as generous, charitable, and altruistic—but they are not these things. They are frightened.

In other words, five-sensory individuals may see an act as compassionate that multisensory individuals know may not be. The difference between a compassionate action and a fearful action is intention. Individuals who are pursuing external power are not interested in their intentions. They do not discriminate between intentions that they think they hold (such as helping those less fortunate), hidden intentions that they may or may not realize that they hold (such as creating a self-image of kindness, generosity, or philanthropy), and the real, beneath-everything-else intention that motivates their giving (manipulating and controlling circumstances in order to feel safe and valuable). Individuals who create authentic power strive to know their intention each moment.

Five-sensory humans confuse compassion with sentimentality. They submerge themselves in cozy feelings that they think are loving experiences. For example, they melt when they see pictures of cuddly children and infants. They love images of couples running hand-in-hand through surf and paintings of quaint and homey cottages in perfect evening light where all is as it should be. These are not experiences of compassion but attempts to escape the emotional challenges of the Earth school. Compassion is an aware, fully present state. Sentimentality is absence from your life, a denial of the difficult experiences of frightened parts of your personality. It is a disconnected, fear-based fantasy. Compassion is intimate and real.

The Lakota Indians of North America say that the hurt of one is the hurt of all and the honor of one is the honor of all. We can transport this wisdom into the vocabulary of authentic power by saying that the pain of one is the pain of all and the joy of one is the joy of all. We feel the pain of others, and they feel ours. We feel the joy of others, and they feel ours. Frightened parts of one personality resonate with the experiences of frightened parts of other personalities. If our parent has left the Earth school, we empathize with others who have had similar experiences. Our common suffering creates a sense of shared intimacy. In the same way, loving parts of one personality resonate with the experiences of loving parts of other personalities. For example, if we have experienced the healing power of forgiveness, we empathize with others who have walked that same path. We understand and appreciate them, and they understand and appreciate us.

This natural ability to recognize the experiences of others as our own and feel close to those individuals as a result is not compassion. For example, drug addicts empathize with one another. They share common experiences, but the sense of comfort with one another that results does not help them become healthy. On the contrary, it supports them in remaining addicted. Individuals who see themselves as victims (such as drug addicts) resonate with others who also see themselves as victims. They sympathize, empathize, and pity one another, but that is not compassion.

When I was in the army I felt more comfortable with fellow Special Forces (Green Beret) soldiers than with others. We empathized and sympathized, but we had no compassion no matter how much we felt that we cared about one another. Our mission demanded denial of the humanity, sensitivity, and suffering of our enemies; required inhumanity and insensitivity from us; and elevated our suffering to heroism. Compassion changes all this. It obliterates the distinction between allies and adversaries, and only fellow students in the Earth school remain. Compassion opens your heart and your eyes. Care for others replaces fear of others. The pain and joy of others help you to create authentic power and to help others create authentic power. You see the sources of their pain (frightened parts of the personality) and joy (loving parts of the personality), and you care enough to help them challenge and heal the frightened parts and cultivate the loving parts, if they choose.

This is a very different dynamic than caretaking, creating a self-pleasing self-image, and manipulating others with actions that appear to be compassionate. It is different than remaining imprisoned in shared experiences of powerlessness. It is using your understanding of the experiences of others to support them in creating authentic power. It is caring about them. My experiences in the army, for example, help me to communicate with those who wear uniforms and carry weapons, such as police officers, but that ability is not compassion. They help me relate to anyone who serves the public in uniform, such as firefighters and people in the coast guard, but that ability is not compassion either. Caring about others enough to use my understanding to help them is compassion.

Comfort in the company of those with similar experiences is the glue that binds individuals into larger collectives such as cultures, nations, religions, races, and the sexes, and into smaller collectives such as professional, trade, and social organizations. The white-only, no-Jews country club is an example. It creates countless affinities between individuals who share common experiences as diverse as parenthood, stock trading, and plumbing. It is the Universal Law of Attraction at work. Generically, there are only two energies—love and fear—and the Universal Law of Attraction continually brings love together with love and fear together with fear. It brings those who are challenging their fear into the company of others who are also challenging their fear, and those who are cultivating love together with others who are cultivating love.

Challenging a frightened part of your personality (which also cultivates a loving part of your personality) creates compassion. It changes your experiences of yourself and your experiences of others at the same time. The less you judge yourself, the less you judge others. The more you appreciate yourself, the more you appreciate others. When you love yourself, you love others. Compassion for yourself and compassion for others are two sides of the same coin. One side is your interactions with frightened and loving parts of your personality. The other side is your interactions with frightened and loving parts of other personalities.

The loving parts of your personality are compassionate, and the frightened parts are not. If you do not choose between them, a frightened part of your personality will choose for you and you will not experience compassion, no matter how compassionate your actions may appear to others. Choosing to act with the intention of a loving part of your personality while you are feeling the painful sensations of a frightened part of your personality, observing its judgmental thoughts, and seeing its destructive intention creates authentic power. It also creates compassionate words and deeds. In other words, compassionate words and actions require conscious choices. Shouting when you are angry is an unconscious choice. Having sex when you feel the need and a willing partner appears is an unconscious choice. So are smoking when you crave a cigarette, drinking when you need a drink, and gambling when you feel the impulse. Compassionate words and actions are not obsessive, compulsive, or addictive. They are appropriate.

You cannot be compassionate with one person and not be compassionate with all people any more than you can be compassionate with all people and not be compassionate with yourself. Compassion has no exclusions (including you) or exceptions (including you). It opens, unlocks, and removes barriers. It is care without fear, without agendas, attachments, or expectations. Compassion cannot be wished, affirmed, visualized, or prayed into being any more than a farmer can wish, affirm, visualize, or pray a crop into being. He can choose the crop that he wants to harvest, but that is not enough. He must prepare the ground, plant the seeds, water and feed them, and pull the weeds. If you want to harvest compassion, you must create authentic power.

At some point in the creation of authentic power your endeavors become real to you. You realize that your emotional awareness and responsible choices are affecting the very substance of your life—your ability to live outside of the control of the frightened parts of your personality and to create a life of love. When you realize, and truly realize, that allowing the frightened parts of your personality to do as they choose is more painful than challenging them, the courage that challenging them requires begins to be replaced with the gratification of challenging them and choosing responsibly instead of reacting irresponsibly. You begin to create different consequences for yourself and others. You no longer change in order to please others, be accepted, or make yourself feel valuable or safe. You change because you want to change, because you are no longer willing to be controlled by the frightened parts of your personality. You change because you no longer want to experience the pain of the frightened parts of your personality and the pain of the consequences that they create.

You attract others who are doing the same, and you also see the depth of the pain of others—the pain of powerlessness and the pain of the destructive consequences that attempting to avoid it has created—because you experience that pain yourself. This is the birth of compassion.

You know how difficult it is to challenge and heal a frightened part of your personality, and because of that you know how difficult it is for others as well. You also see the freedom that you are creating within yourself, and you want to share with others how to create that freedom—how to use their experiences, including their painful experiences, to become masters of their own lives. You taste the fruits of your efforts, and you see that no one else could have given them to you. Then you see how desperately others are looking for someone or something to provide them meaning and purpose, fulfillment and joy, and how futile that search is.

That is when the need to teach, fix, impress, convert, or caretake disappears. That is when the pursuit of external power loses its attraction. Humbleness, clarity, forgiveness, and Love fill your life; all that remains are the intentions of your soul, and you use them to guide you, creating at each moment with an empowered heart without attachment to the outcome.

That is the way to create compassion that continues between moments of inspiration, that endures after the sermon is over, that guides you without fail through the most difficult experiences and transforms them into some of the most rewarding.

26

Compassion Guidelines

Compassion is being moved to and by acts of the heart. Only loving parts of the personality are motivated by the heart. The frightened parts of the personality are oriented differently. Possible acts of the heart are limitless. Opportunities for them arise each moment, and each is uniquely defined by time and circumstance. Your creativity is without limit, and so, therefore, are the ways that you can act with compassion.

Practicing the compassion guidelines will create compassion in you. Imagine following them when you are alone with your thoughts, and follow them when you are with your spiritual partners and with those who do not know about spiritual partnership. If you are not sure how to challenge a frightened part of your personality or you do not see a compassionate response in the moment, follow them. Then follow them again.

- **CHANGE MY PERSPECTIVE from fearful to loving (choose to see myself and others in a loving or appreciative way).**

Changing your perspective from fearful to loving is the operative dynamic in the creation of authentic power. It is the shift from anxiety to appreciation and from pain to joy. You cannot change your emotions at will, but you can choose what you will do when your emotions come. You can re-act (act again as you have previously and unconsciously) or respond (act differently, consciously choose another intention, create anew). When you are angry, depressed, jealous, thinking critical thoughts, or having any of the familiar, painful experiences of frightened parts of your personality, you can choose to shift your perceptions to those of a loving part of your personality.

The frightened parts of your personality always experience fearful perceptions, and the loving parts always enjoy loving perceptions. They continually offer you the fundamental choice of the Earth school—love or fear. Will you accept, wallow in, and drown in the perceptions of a frightened part of your personality, fortifying yourself in its familiar painful experiences, or will you acknowledge them, feel them, and challenge them by shifting your attention to other perspectives, other possible ways of understanding, and other intentions? When you choose to remain in the experiences and distorted perceptions of frightened parts of your personality, you pursue external power. You create authentic power when you use your volition to explore elsewhere and make the healthiest choices that you can, even while the frightened parts of your personality call magnetically to you.

Sometimes the Universe gives you the experience of shifting to a loving perspective without effort on your part—a grace-filled change of experience from fear to love. You may have had such an experience. For example, Linda and I were settling into our seats for a flight home after a long trip. We were pleased to have an empty seat between us. It gave us a place to put our books, notes, and snacks and to stretch out. Just before the doors closed a disheveled man came down the aisle toward us. He stopped beside Linda and showed her his ticket for the empty seat. Linda offered him her aisle seat and moved over to sit next to me. His clothes were rumpled, he was unshaven, his hair was unkempt, and he smelled of alcohol.

I could feel Linda's concern. I was concerned about having him next to us for the long flight, also. We sat silently through takeoff and the first twenty minutes. When a flight attendant came by he ordered a bourbon although it was early morning. Linda usually enjoys speaking with fellow travelers, but this time she remained quiet. I saw her thinking (or feeling) as she pondered the person beside her. Then to my surprise she asked him, "Where are you from?" He looked at her indirectly and said softly, "I have just buried my daughter."

His simple words opened my heart, and I saw that they deeply touched Linda also. She became available and interested instead of judgmental and distant. Gently she asked him more questions, and slowly his story emerged. By the time we arrived at the airport, we had become friends. He intended to take a taxi home, but when we realized how close he lived, we offered to drop him off. The last time we saw him he was waving us good-bye. I did not hear Linda's conversation with him through most of the flight, but I know she spoke gently to him about frightened and loving parts of the personality and helped him, as well as she could, to see his grief and pain as experiences coming from parts of his personality that can be challenged and healed.

Practicing this guideline will help you remember to look for ways to shift your perspective from fearful to loving. When you are waiting impatiently in an express checkout line, for example, and the person at the front of the line is searching for her checkbook although checks are not allowed, and then slowly writing a check for a basketful of groceries although only a few items are allowed, it will remind you to ask yourself if you have ever done the same thing accidentally (or intentionally). Does she remind you of your grandmother, or your favorite neighbor? Would anyone you love or care for perhaps do the same thing without realizing that others are waiting?

Look for ways to let a new perspective dissolve your fear. Allow yourself to become one who, at this time and in this place, appreciates instead of judges, loves instead of fears, and creates authentic power.

- **RELEASE ANY DISTANCE I feel from anyone.**

When you feel distant from others, a frightened part of your personality is active. There are as many ways to create distance from people as there are experiences of frightened parts of your personality, for example, jealousy, resentment, anger, need to please, and feeling entitled, overwhelmed, inadequate, or impatient. All of them are opportunities to challenge and heal frightened parts of your personality and cultivate loving parts. You will know that the frightened part of your personality no longer controls you when you feel close again (or for the first time) with someone else.

In the last century the Swiss psychologist Carl Jung illuminated a way for anyone to discover frightened parts of his or her personality in certain circumstances and to experience them (although he did not use the term "frightened parts of the personality," and he wrote for psychoanalysts). What you do not want to see in yourself (a frightened part of your personality) you "project" onto the world and see outside of you. You never like it when you see it there. Jung called this dynamic *projection.*

In other words, what you find too painful or shameful to acknowledge in yourself you see in others, and you do not like it in them. If you think of yourself as caring, for example, but frightened parts of your personality do not care about others, you will find individuals who do not care about others repulsive. They may or may not be caring people. The important thing is your painful emotional experience when you see (or think you see) lack of caring in another.

The degree of repulsion that you feel is a measure of how much you do not want to recognize in yourself what you think you see in another. If you really do not want to see something in yourself, you really will not like it when you see it in someone else. The most rigid, righteous, virulent crusades, such as those against homosexuality and prostitution, are examples of projection. As many crusaders have discovered, they are attracted to what they hate, and they are so terrified by their attraction that they cannot consider the possibility of it in themselves. The more they battle what they hate outside of themselves, the stronger their attraction to it becomes. Eventually, they find themselves doing what they most despise, such as having sex with a prostitute.

You can see for yourself whether or not you project parts of your personality onto others, and give yourself the experience of releasing any distance that you feel from them in the process. The next time you instantly dislike someone you just met or have seen only from a distance, notice what you do not like about that person. Make a note of each thing that repulses you. Be specific. For example, "He is arrogant. He is impolite. He is selfish." Then look for these behaviors in you.

At first it may seem impossible that you could be similar in any way to the person you find so unlikable. Be persistent. Eventually you will find in yourself exactly what you do not like in him or her. When you do, your judgments will melt away. Like recognizing in yourself the person who slows your progress through the checkout line, you will recognize in yourself the person who irritates, annoys, or angers you, and the distance between you and that person will disappear at the same time. You will understand him. You will know his experiences because you share them. Instead of a hateful object, you will see him as one who has frightened parts of his personality that are like the frightened parts of yours.

Shortly after I met Linda I found myself annoyed at what I perceived to be her whining. I understood projection, but I could not imagine how it could apply to me in this case. Green Berets do not whine. I did many things I did not want to admit, but whining, in my opinion, was not one of them. However, Linda's whining (or my perception of her whining) continued to annoy me, so I began to look for whining in me. One afternoon when Linda suggested that I might be doing something that I could not imagine myself doing (something other than whining), the last word of my answer to her ("I do not!") slid down the scale and then back up again almost an octave. It was a first-class whine. I heard myself whining! I *knew* that I would if I listened carefully enough, and I did. Discovering a frightened part of my personality that I could not imagine existing was a liberating experience for me.

Whether or not the person you push away is actually the way that you think she is, a painful emotional charge tells you that a frightened part of your personality is active. If you are honest, for example, noticing dishonesty in another will not create an emotional reaction in you. You will see the frightened part of her personality that is dishonest and act accordingly (for example, not give her the keys to your house). If you are also dishonest, or not willing to admit that you are not always in integrity, you will judge her, blame her, avoid her, gossip about her, etc., for being dishonest. In other words, recognizing a frightened part of your personality in the personality of another individual is not a projection. Reacting emotionally to it is.

• BE PRESENT while others are speaking (not preparing replies, judging, etc.).

When the person you are with does not command your attention, you lose power. Being present to others is not a communication skill. It is required in order to enter your life consciously. When you are with someone you are not paying attention to, for example, thinking of a reply or of what you should be doing somewhere else or feeling that he is not worthy of your attention, you step into an emptiness of daydreams and preoccupations. Interactions with fellow students in the Earth school are the substance of your curriculum in it. When you are not present with others, you cannot see opportunities that the Universe provides you to find the roots of your pain and your joy. You sit beside a well, thirsty. Water is there, but you cannot see it. Some people spend their entire lives thirsty.

My adopted Sioux uncle told me, "Nephew, always listen respectfully when someone speaks, even if you think what he is saying is nonsense." He was not interested in flattering people. He was committed to creating a life of power. You can leave a conversation without letting your attention leave it first. There are no casual or random interactions. You and those you encounter are fellow souls, learning lessons of power, responsibility, wisdom, or love.

Daydreams, regrets, and anticipation are experiences of frightened parts of your personality that cannot fulfill you no matter how many of them you have. Are your most meaningful memories of vacating, ignoring fellow souls, or retreating into your thoughts? Or are they of souls who gave you the gift of their presence and received the gift of yours?

Power exists only in the present moment. Savor each moment, not by grasping it, but by expanding it.

27

Conscious Communications and Actions

CONSCIOUS COMMUNICATIONS AND ACTIONS—STRIVING TO MAKE ALL MY INTERACTIONS CONSCIOUS AND LOVING

Creating authentic power encompasses the totality of your life. It envelopes all of your experiences, includes all of your emotions and thoughts, and reveals all of your intentions. No interaction, person, circumstance, or experience is excluded. Your whole life complete serves the creation of authentic power. Nothing is too big (such as a terminal illness), too important (such as the attack on the World Trade Center), or too monumental (such as global economic dysfunction) to be excluded. Nothing is too small (such as a jealous thought), too insignificant (such as a fleeting hunch), or too unimportant (such as a gift for a child) not to be included.

Attempting to create authentic power without using everything in your life is like trying to swim without water. You can imagine swimming, picture it, read about it, be inspired by it, and even practice moving your arms and head as though you were swimming, but without water you cannot swim. You cannot swim on a wet floor. You cannot swim in a shallow stream. You need to immerse yourself in water, submerge yourself totally, enter the water completely. When you set the intention to swim, that intention will lead you directly to water. When you set the intention to create authentic power, that intention will take you directly to interactions with others.

Creating authentic power is different from every previous spiritual, religious, and self-help endeavor. Authentic power makes no sense (and has no use) to five-sensory humans who pray to the universe to help them defeat enemies, ask deities for advantages, and manipulate and control circumstances and others to survive. Creating authentic power uproots every part of your personality that values your experiences more than the experiences of others, your well-being more than the well-being of others, your life more than the lives of others. It transforms your experiences into a learning adventure, a sea of compassion that continually offers you opportunities to swim (create authentic power) or drown (pursue external power).

You swim when you create your experiences consciously, choose love instead of fear, and fulfill your sacred contract with the Universe. You drown when you continue to create as you have in the past (unconsciously in fear), encounter destructive consequences (painful karma), and attempt to escape the pain of powerlessness by pursuing external power.

Until you learn to swim, events and circumstances overwhelm you. You long for what you do not have and fear to lose what you have. Frightened parts of your personality determine your perceptions, experiences, and intentions. You fear life and you fear death. You pray for Divine intervention without understanding its purpose—to assist you in living a life of love, gratitude, and fulfillment, not to relieve you of the work that you were born to do.

Multisensory perception illuminates a higher order of reasoning and justice. It reveals relationships between the outer world and the inner world that five-sensory humans do not see. Five-sensory humans believe that their emotional experiences are caused by external circumstances. Multisensory humans know that their emotional experiences are independent of external circumstances. Five-sensory humans see their lives as obstacle courses or random impositions of a cruel universe. Multisensory humans see each life as a journey through an educational environment (the Earth school) that is designed for the benefit of souls learning to grow spiritually through the choices that their personalities make.

(Most) five-sensory humans strive to make their interactions conscious and loving when appropriate. Multisensory humans in pursuit of authentic power make all of their interactions conscious and loving because they long for wholeness and intend to create it. They refuse to be controlled any longer by anger, jealousy, vengefulness, resentment, and rage. They take seriously Gandhi's challenge to be the change they want to see, and they know that the influence of their choices extends far beyond the domain of the five senses.

Five-sensory humans think interactions that remove, abate, or minimize suffering are loving. Multisensory humans know the issue is more complex. Is it loving to imprison a criminal? (No one wants to go to prison.) Is it loving to set him free? (He could attack someone else.) Is it loving to keep an employee who will not challenge his drug addiction? (He will buy drugs while he has money.) Is it loving to fire him? (His family needs his support.)

Five-sensory humans distinguish loving interactions from those that are not by circumstance. Multisensory humans distinguish them by intention. If you seek revenge, imprisoning a criminal is not loving. If you strive to protect others without judging the criminal, imprisoning him is loving. If you fear an employee who is addicted and need to impose your will upon him in order to feel safe and worthy, firing him is not loving. If you care for him, his family, and his health, firing him is loving.

Conscious and loving interactions are desirable to five-sensory humans. They are essential to multisensory humans who create authentic power. Transforming unconscious and unloving interactions into conscious and loving interactions challenges every frightened part of your personality and cultivates every loving part.

Creating authentic power combines spiritual growth and creating conscious and loving communications and actions into a single endeavor that is your life. For example, feeding hungry individuals with a second agenda to sell them your belief system is not loving. Feeding them because they are hungry is loving. Caring for the sick in order to make yourself feel safe and worthy (superior, righteous, doing the right thing, etc.) is not loving. Caring for them because they need help is loving. Only you can know your intention at the moment that you speak or act, and your intention (love or fear) creates unambiguous consequences. There are no blurry lines.

When Gandhi visited the Pashtun people near the Khyber Pass in what was then the North-West Frontier Province of India, his friends cautioned him, "These people are fighters." "I, too, am a fighter," replied Gandhi. "I want to teach them how to fight without violence—how to fight without fear." "Are you afraid?" he asked them. "Why else would you be carrying guns?" They stared at him. No one had addressed them in this way. "I have no fear," Gandhi continued. "That is why I am unarmed." At the end of the interaction a tall Pashtun, Khan Abdul Ghaffar Khan, put down his rifle, and others followed. This giant of a man became a dedicated companion to Gandhi, accompanying him (unarmed) on many of Gandhi's courageous challenges to policies of the British government. Khan Abdul Ghaffar Khan appears in many pictures with Gandhi, always easy to identify, towering above those around him. This interaction was loving.

Creating conscious and loving interactions makes you a spiritual activist like Gandhi—unrestrained by fear and free of the need to punish villains. It enables you, like Gandhi, like King, like all those who decline to hate in a world of hatred, like all those who love adversaries and allies alike, to cocreate a world that reflects the intentions of the soul.

The creation of authentic power brings you into the world, not away from it. It connects you with fellow souls, not separates you from them. Your interactions with others are the bottom line of your spiritual development. You cannot become spiritually evolved and remain in the control of frightened parts of your personality, because frightened parts of your personality create unconscious and unloving interactions. Whatever you call your path, it is not spiritual if your interactions are not becoming more conscious and more loving. Your interactions with others show you where you have more work to do. They also show you the distance you have traveled.

Creating authentic power produces conscious and loving interactions, and creating conscious and loving interactions is necessary to creating authentic power. Commitment, courage, compassion, and conscious communications and actions merge in the creation of an authentically empowered life.

28

Conscious Communications and Actions Guidelines

The demeanor of an old acquaintance surprised me. Several years earlier he had appeared lighthearted, innocent, and cheerful. Now he was troubled and sullen. He had inherited a small house, he told me, moved into it, and rented his home. Now his renters were months behind in their payments, vandalizing his house, and enjoying free utilities because the accounts were still in his name. "There is nothing I can do," he explained. "Eviction in my state is a slow and expensive process. Meanwhile, I am seeing my house damaged, losing rental income, and paying the mortgage on the house and their utilities."

He had traveled to several countries as a volunteer missionary with his church. He saw himself as generous and kind before this experience, but he was not prepared for the unexpected emotions, thoughts, and fantasies that flooded through him now. They troubled him more than the financial hardship he faced, confusing him and causing him to question his goodness, his values, and his intentions.

The Spiritual Partnership Guidelines are designed for precisely this kind of situation (they are designed for every kind of situation). The conscious communications and actions guidelines are a shorthand checklist for creating authentic power. The following are some examples of how they might be applied to my acquaintance's circumstances. As you read, imagine how they might apply to your own.

- **CONSULT MY INTUITION.**

Intuition is access to compassion and wisdom that is beyond what we are able to give one another. It is communication with nonphysical guides and Teachers, whose only interest is your spiritual growth. The first part of accessing intuition is to ask a question. The second part is to listen for the answer. The answer will always come, although perhaps not in the way or at the time that you expect. There are many ways that my acquaintance could have approached his tenants—directly, through an attorney, delicately, bluntly, etc. When you ask, "What would be the most appropriate way to do what I want to do?" (in this case, move the tenants out of his house), you will always have insights.

Your answer might come while you are in the shower, out for a walk, or driving to work. It may not be what you want to hear. Answers that come from your intuition will often surprise you. Your intellect will always rationalize what you want to do.

Intuitive insights are not directives, instructions, or commandments. Your nonphysical Teachers will not tell you what to do. They will lead you to the full scope and depth of your creative capacity, help you see options that you have not thought about, and consider the consequences that each will create. Only you can decide how you will use your will to shape energy into matter, what karma you will create. Responsibility for your choices is always yours alone, no matter whom you consult in the process of making them, including nonphysical Teachers.

- **CHOOSE MY INTENTION before I speak or act.**

Intentions are causes that create effects. Choosing an intention is the fundamental creative act. An intention is the reason, or motivation, for doing what you do. Every action has an intention, and every intention comes from a loving part of the personality or a frightened part. The same action can have different intentions. For example, the motivation for making a lot of money might be to buy stylish clothing or a beautiful car that will attract attention and recognition, or it might be to pay school expenses for a child. The first intention is the pursuit of external power. The second creates authentic power.

When you chose your intention before you speak or act, you choose the consequences that your words or action will create. If you do not choose your intentions consciously, you will choose them unconsciously (frightened parts of your personality will choose them for you). You can always recognize the consequences of unconscious choices (choices made outside your awareness by frightened parts of your personality) because they hurt when you encounter them. The more you explore your intentions, the more you will see that no matter how many options you appear to have, you actually have only two—love and fear. Loving intentions create authentic power.

If you are not certain of your intention, ask yourself before you speak or act, "What is my motivation?" You will not be alone in your assessment. This is a fail-safe way to consult intuition. If your intention is anything except harmony, cooperation, sharing, or reverence for Life—if it is not to care for others, support others, and contribute constructively to Life without second agendas, it will be to manipulate and control (pursue external power).

My acquaintance could have asked himself (each time) before he spoke with his tenants, "What is my motivation?" and used his painful experiences with them to create authentic power by choosing a loving intention each time he discovered that he was about to speak or act with an intention that was not loving.

• ACT FROM THE HEALTHIEST PART OF MY PERSONAL-
ITY that I can access (rather than caretaking, fixing, teaching,
judging, blaming, gossiping, etc.).

Choosing to act from a loving part of your personality while
you are feeling the painful sensations of a frightened part of
your personality is the moment of traction on the spiritual path.
Choosing to act from the healthiest part of your personality that
you can find instead of one that is less healthy is the step that
stretches you beyond the limitations of the frightened parts of
your personality, the moment when authentic power is created,
the instant when spiritual growth occurs. All of this depends
upon your choice.

My acquaintance was shocked by the powerful and painful
emotions that swept through him and the images that appeared to
him when he interacted with his tenants or thought about them.
His self-image as a generous and kind person could not accom-
modate experiences of rage, helplessness, humiliation, vengefulness, and then rage again. Cycling from one painful experience of
powerlessness to another, he spiraled downward into anger, confusion, and guilt. He reproached himself for his violent thoughts
and fantasies and at the same time was attracted to them.

My acquaintance had discovered frightened parts of his personality. Most individuals do not think that they are capable
of murderous rage, intentionally inflicting pain, and wishing
others ill. All of us are. "My lawyer tells me these tenants are professionals," he explained. "They do this often, and they know how
to use the law. All I can do is wait." While he waited he smoldered,
then broke into anger, then rage, and then felt guilty for having
these experiences.

Five-sensory humans see these circumstances as unfortunate. Multisensory humans see them as learning opportunities.
My acquaintance's violent fantasies revealed to him frightened

parts of his personality that, had they remained unconscious, would have created painful consequences. They gave him advance notice of what those parts planned to do—and would do—unless he chose otherwise. This is the purpose of temptation. A temptation is a dress rehearsal for a negative karmic event. Temptations allow you to experience and heal negativity within your own sphere of energy before it spills over into the energy spheres of others (such as my acquaintance's tenants). They are gracious gifts from the compassionate and wise Universe that allow you to grow spiritually without harming others or yourself.

My acquaintance's troublesome tenants continued to provide him (when we spoke last) opportunities to experience and challenge frightened parts of his personality by choosing to interact with them from the healthiest parts of his personality instead of the least healthy. They are his allies in the creation of authentic power.

• **SPEAK PERSONALLY AND SPECIFICALLY** rather than generally and abstractly (use "I" statements rather than "we" or "you" statements).

My acquaintance told me, explaining his experiences as if they were the experiences of everyone, "We are afraid of what we will do when we are angry." What he meant was "I am afraid of what I will do when I am angry." Speaking in general terms about others instead of in specific terms about yourself obscures the frightened parts of your personality and dilutes your experience of them. Creating authentic power requires feeling the full power of these destructive and painful aspects of your personality and challenging them while you do.

I learned from my adopted Sioux uncle that the Lakota language is not always translatable into English, but there are parts of it that are very understandable and powerful to English speakers. For example, when an individual assembles people for a gathering or creates an event, he states his name and says *"he me yelo*" (hay may' yeah-low) at the conclusion of it. If I were Lakota, I would say at the end of each event on authentic power that I create, "Gary Zukav *he me yelo.*" This means, "I am Gary Zukav. I am responsible for what has happened here. If anyone has questions about it, come to me." When you speak personally and specifically instead of abstractly and generally, you do the same thing. You recognize your responsibility for your words and actions.

As you create authentic power you become the authority in your life. You take responsibility for what you choose and do not choose, for what you pay attention to and what you do not, for what you create.

• **RELEASE ATTACHMENT TO THE OUTCOME (trust the Universe). If I find myself attached, begin again with Commitment, Courage, Compassion.**

The highest priority for five-sensory humans is manipulating and controlling circumstances (the pursuit of external power). For example, my acquaintance was attached to evicting his non-paying tenants as quickly as possible, minimizing damage to his house, and renting it again. The highest priority for multisensory humans is growing spiritually (creating authentic power). This difference in priorities changes their experiences and the consequences that they create.

Five-sensory humans seek solutions in order to feel safe and valuable. Multisensory humans learn about themselves in order to create authentic power. A five-sensory human sees circumstances to maintain or change. A multisensory human sees opportunities to grow spiritually. They both strive to keep their eyes on a ball. The ball for five-sensory humans is a physical goal. The ball for multisensory humans is authentic power. When you find yourself attached to an outcome, you are focusing on the wrong ball. Attachment to an outcome that will make you feel valuable or safe tells you that you are pursuing external power.

When you create authentic power your understanding of what

needs to be done in the moment—evicting tenants, finding a new job, learning to say no without anger, learning to say yes without pleasing, and so on—becomes more accurate, your actions more effective, and you create constructive and joyful consequences instead of destructive and painful consequences. Every circumstance provides you an opportunity to choose anew, to step into a different and healthy perspective of what you need to do, why you are doing it, and how to do it.

Here is a micro-checklist for creating authentic power:

• TRUST. The compassion and wisdom of the Universe are visible and available for experimentation everywhere, in all circumstances, at all times. Every circumstance activates emotional currents—produces pleasant or painful sensations, judgmental or appreciative thoughts, and constructive or destructive intentions. Each circumstance provides a new opportunity to consult intuition, use emotional awareness, choose responsibly, and align your personality with your soul. In youth and old age, health and illness, wealth and poverty new circumstances continue to appear like grass in the spring—karma continues to unfold—and each brings a new opportunity to create authentic power. Once you see this, you will not forget it and will not fear to lose it.

  That is trust.

• RELAX. Frightened parts of the personality run from the pain of powerlessness into difficult emotions, obsessive thoughts, compulsive activities, and addictive behaviors. Their sense of safety depends upon external circumstances, external circumstances change, and therefore they continually need to manipulate and control them. The frightened parts of your personality are terrified of dying, yet from the multisensory perspective, you cannot be annihilated. Once you realize that, the rest is merely experience. The more you create authentic power, the more you see that every circumstance offers you an opportunity to choose anew, to create authentic power again. Then you can say to yourself, "The Universe is my cocreator," and relax into the cocreation. Relax into your partnership with the Universe. Relax into the eternal present moment. Relax into your life and everything that is in it.

- DO YOUR BEST. My acquaintance talked to his tenants, consulted with the city, and hired an attorney, but he did not trust the Universe and so he could not relax and do his best. He intended to accomplish his goal (eviction) but not to create authentic power in the process. His painful emotions appeared as obstacles to him, potent distractions from his goal instead of messages from his soul to help him grow spiritually (a frightened part of your personality is active or a loving part of your personality is active). When you trust the Universe and are relaxed, you can do your best. Until then, you can't. My acquaintance could have (accurately) viewed his painful experiences as gifts from the Universe helping him to locate and heal frightened parts of his personality in order to move into his full potential. Using your experiences to create authentic power is always the best that you can do, and nothing more is asked of you.

- ENJOY YOURSELF. When you see the wisdom and compassion of the Universe, relax into your life, and do your best; there is nothing more that you can do. Then take your hands off the steering wheel. Let your nonphysical guides and Teachers do their part. Let the Universe do its part. You cannot know how the Universe works or fathom its compassion and wisdom, and you do not need to know. You need only trust, relax, do your best, and enjoy yourself.

29

The Evolving Guidelines

The Spiritual Partnership Guidelines are evolving.

They will evolve for you, too, as your understanding of authentic power and your commitment to creating it deepen.

Print out the Spiritual Partnership Guidelines from www.seatofthesoul.com and tape them to your mirrors and fridge. Take them to work and keep a copy in your purse or wallet. Don't be shy about referring to them often.

Practice the Spiritual Partnership Guidelines at home, with family, at work, and at school, long enough to know them by heart as well as mind, long enough to experiment with them again and again, long enough to experience creating authentic power often, and then draw upon your experiences to see if you can contribute constructively to them.

Then experiment some more.

SPIRITUAL PARTNERSHIP GUIDELINES

Commitment—Making My Spiritual Growth (Creating Authentic Power) My Highest Priority

- **Focus on what I can learn about myself** all the time, especially from my reactions (such as anger, fear, jealousy, resentment, and impatience), instead of judging or blaming others or myself.
- **Pay attention to my emotions** by feeling the physical sensations in my energy centers (such as my chest, solar plexus, and throat areas).
- **Pay attention to my thoughts** (such as judging, analyzing, comparing, daydreaming, planning my reply, etc., or thoughts of gratitude, appreciation, contentment, openness to Life, etc.).
- **Pay attention to my intention** (such as blaming, judging, needing to be right, seeking admiration, escaping into thoughts (intellectualizing), trying to convince, etc., or cooperating, sharing, creating harmony, and revering Life).

Courage—Stretching Myself Beyond the Limited Perspectives of the Frightened Parts of My Personality

- **Take responsibility** for my feelings, experiences, and actions (no blaming).
- **Practice integrity at all times** (often requires action, such as speaking when frightened parts of my personality don't want to speak and not speaking when they feel compelled to speak).
- **Say or do what is most difficult** (sharing what I notice, if appropriate, when someone speaks or acts from a frightened

part of his or her personality; sharing about myself what I am frightened to say and know that I need to say).

Compassion—Seeing Myself and Others as Souls Who Sometimes Have Frightened Parts of Their Personalities Active

- **Change my perspective** from fearful to loving (choose to see myself and others in a loving or appreciative way).
- **Release any distance** I feel from anyone.
- **Be present** while others are speaking (not preparing replies, judging, etc.).

Conscious Communications and Actions—Striving to Make All My Interactions Conscious and Loving

- **Consult my intuition.**
- **Choose my intention** before I speak or act.
- **Act from the healthiest part of my personality** that I can access (rather than caretaking, fixing, teaching, judging, blaming, gossiping, etc.).
- **Speak personally and specifically** rather than generally and abstractly (use "I" statements rather than "we" or "you" statements).
- **Release attachment to the outcome** (trust the Universe). If I find myself attached, begin again with Commitment, Courage, Compassion.

30
Soul Summary

SPIRITUAL PARTNERSHIPS—
PUTTING THEM INTO ACTION

Now come the action steps, the life-changing movements, the transformation of energy into matter, possibility into experience. The Spiritual Partnership Guidelines cannot create authentic power or spiritual partnerships, but applying them does. There are countless ways to create authentic power because there are countless circumstances in your life. Each moment brings another, and each offers numerous possibilities to create authentic power and the potential of spiritual partnerships in numerous ways.

Each drop in an ocean, flake in a snowy storm, and circumstance in your life is unique, perfect, and transient. This is the context in which authentic power is created. Let your intuition, experience, and the support of your spiritual partners combine to show you ways to apply the Spiritual Partnership Guidelines, or experiment with applying them, in each circumstance.

Some helpful suggestions follow, but who can provide you more than suggestions once you understand that you alone are responsible for the consequences that you create in your life? Relax into the process. Enjoy the process. Most important, begin the process.

31

Spiritual Partnership in Action 1

Frightened parts of your personality are closed systems of emotions, thoughts, perceptions, and intentions. They are not interested in changing. Until you challenge them, they will remain in control of you. Challenging a frightened part of your personality requires the conscious application of your will while the frightened part is active—while you feel the need to shout, lash out, withdraw emotionally, please or dominate, and so on. Looking inward at this part of your personality—experiencing the painful physical sensations in your energy centers, noticing your thoughts, and observing your intention—instead of reacting is the first challenge to it.

The choice to challenge a frightened part of your personality will not come from the frightened part. For example, when you are angry, a frightened part of your personality intends to remain angry. It will not choose otherwise. That is your job. If you are not willing to challenge a frightened part of your personality, it remains unchallenged and your behaviors and inner experiences remain unchanged. You do not grow spiritually. You use an opportunity to create authentic power to pursue external power instead.

Recognizing this allows you to take the first step in supporting a spiritual partner when frightened parts of her personality are active and allows you to be supported by her when frightened parts of your personality are active. The first step is willingness to look at the part of your personality that is seething, roaring, erupting, or exploding in you. Without that first step, there can be no second step. Therefore, when a spiritual partner is reacting (in the control of a frightened part of her personality), or you think that she is, the first step is to ask:

"Are you willing to challenge this?"

There are many ways to articulate this question, but the question always remains the same: Are you willing in this moment to examine your interior experiences? If the answer is no, you can go no further. Ignoring her answer and imposing yourself is the pursuit of external power. If the answer is yes, experiment with appropriate questions, such as:

"Are you feeling anything in your body?"

Help your spiritual partner locate specific physical sensations in the vicinity of her chest, solar plexus, throat, and other energy centers. Remind her to use words such as "stabbing," "aching," "throbbing," "constricted," "relaxed," "warm," and "cold" instead of words such as "sad," "happy," "light," "good," and "bad." Guide her attention to each of her energy centers so that she can become familiar with the sensations in each while the frightened part of her personality is active. The painful sensations that she locates will show her that a frightened part of her personality is active.

"What thoughts are you having?"

Help your spiritual partner become aware of her thoughts. Even if she cannot locate physical sensations in her body, she will be able to notice her thoughts, for example, thoughts that are critical of herself and others or appreciative of herself and others; resentful or grateful; and comparing or contented. Thoughts that are critical, resentful, or comparing, etc., will show her that a frightened part of her personality is active.

If she is still reluctant to acknowledge that a frightened part of her personality is active, use your intuition to find appropriate next steps. For example, you might ask, "If you were in a frightened part of your personality, what would it want to say?" ("I feel you are making me wrong," or "I feel threatened," etc.) You can always ask, "Is that a loving thought or an unloving thought?" The answer will often be evident to her. Use questions that sensitively guide instead of direct or instruct, such as, "Isn't it amazing that when we really look at the thoughts and the perspective of a frightened part of the personality, it becomes so obvious that they don't come from a loving part of the personality? Can you see that?" If the answer is yes, help her to take the next step. For example,

"It is possible to heal this part of your personality by challenging it right now. Would you want to do that?"

If the answer is no, you can go no further. The prerequisite for creating authentic power is the intention to create authentic power. Without it no challenge to frightened parts of the personality is possible no matter how much the vocabulary of authentic power is used and the concepts of authentic power are discussed. If the answer is yes, new possibilities appear. The second step to challenging a frightened part of the personality is to choose anew, create with a different and healthy intention, create constructive consequences instead of the destructive consequences that the intentions of the frightened part of the personality always create.

For example, if your spiritual partner is angry and she habitually withdraws emotionally when she becomes angry, a responsible choice for her (a choice that creates consequences for which she is willing to assume responsibility) would be to remain present. If she habitually shouts when she becomes angry, a responsible choice for her would be to remain silent, or to listen, even if she needs to clinch her fists and force her mouth to remain closed in order to do so.

The most common question that I am asked by students who are beginning to learn authentic power is "What do I do now?": "I am feeling pain in my chest, or throat, or solar plexus area, etc. I know that a frightened part of my personality is active. What do I do now?" Eventually they realize that "What do I do now?" is the eternal question and they alone can answer it.

They have only two options—to challenge the frightened part of the personality that is active or to indulge it—to create with anger, in this case, or with the intention to create constructive consequences even while they are experiencing the pain of powerlessness. The ultimate choice is always between love and fear, between the creation of authentic power and the pursuit of external power. The more your spiritual partner recognizes the painful consequences for herself of pursuing external power and the benefits to herself of creating authentic power, the more incentive she feels to create authentic power. Creating a blissful, loving, healthy future filled with grateful, loving, healthy people instead of a painful, destructive future filled with angry, avaricious, vengeful, or jealous people is a powerful incentive.

Support your spiritual partner in taking this second step, the step that chips away at the walls of her prison, that changes the course of her life, that introduces a conscious choice where previously her choices were unconscious. If she is willing, guide her to it. For example,

"To challenge this part of your personality, how could you see this differently or shift your perspective?"

Each circumstance (opportunity to create authentic power) is unique, and no one understands her circumstance more completely or intimately than your spiritual partner, even while a frightened part of her personality fills her body with pain, distorts her thoughts, and holds destructive intentions. Clothed in her history, formed by her experiences, the opportunity is exquisitely suited to her spiritual growth. She knows the next step better than anyone else. Her nonphysical guides and Teachers can present options to her, illuminate probable consequences, and assist her in using her creative capacity wisely, but she will make the choice that transforms energy into matter, determines the course of her life until her next choice, and brings one of many possible futures into existence.

If you suggest a choice, your interference in her decision becomes a part of your karma. It is the karma of manipulation and control, the karma of external power. It will draw to you others who will attempt to interfere with your decisions. If you help to guide her to her own wisdom with the intention to support her in creating authentic power and without attachment to the outcome, that becomes a part of your karma, and you draw to yourself others who will help to guide you to your own wisdom without attachment to the outcome.

If she decides to challenge the frightened part of her personality, help her to see the power of her decision. Support her in recognizing the role that it plays in the creation of authentic power. Even though she already knows, give her the support of hearing it from a spiritual partner who cares enough about her to be with her while she is feeling the pain of powerlessness and the experiences of a frightened part of her personality surge through her. Reflect her wisdom back to her so that she can see the beauty of it. For example,

"It is such a positive thing to shift your perspective, even just a little bit. It begins the process of healing this part of your personality at a deeper level."

The more sensitivity you bring to your interaction, the more open your spiritual partner is likely to be to your support. Apply the Golden Rule. Would you want a spiritual partner teaching, fixing, caretaking, or trying to manipulate you, or would you want a spiritual partner who brings your attention back to the issues—experiencing and challenging a frightened part of your personality instead of blaming others for its painful experiences or in other ways rationalizing them? Who would most support you in creating authentic power—a friend who sympathizes with you, consoles you, and tries to make you feel better, or a spiritual partner who knows, like you, that the origin of your painful experiences lies within you and the only way to eliminate them is to challenge and heal the inner sources of them; a spiritual partner who will not impose herself but will not be distracted by your tears, anger, withdrawal, and other manipulations from helping you to experience, challenge, and heal the frightened parts of your personality that are tormenting you?

All this is half the process of supporting an individual in creating authentic power—what she experiences.

The other half is what you experience. No matter how sensitive you are or how skilled in following the Spiritual Partnership Guidelines, you cannot support others in creating authentic power without creating it yourself. Creating authentic power is the best support that you can give another who is striving to create authentic power. It requires you to do the things that you are helping her to do. Can you scan your emotional energy centers while you are supporting her? Are you aware of your thoughts and intention while you are supporting him? Are you detached from the outcome of your support? Will you react or respond if the person you are supporting reacts, for example, becomes angry, resentful, or disdainful?

Supporting another in creating authentic power requires caring deeply for that person and holding the intention to create authentic power while you are supporting her. Your interactions may activate frightened parts of your personality that fear her anger, frustration, vengefulness, or jealousy. If that happens, will you respond or react? Does your sense of value and safety depend upon being appreciated? What if she pushes you away? Do you feel superior while you are supporting her, like an insecure teacher might feel toward a student, an insecure professor toward an assistant, or an insecure counselor toward a client? Or do you feel inadequate, unworthy, or unqualified? Are you caretaking, attempting to please, daydreaming, or thinking about the next thing to say? These are experiences of frightened parts of your personality. Will you challenge them while you are supporting her in challenging the frightened parts of her personality?

Supporting others in creating authentic power is a two-way street. It brings your awareness to frightened parts of your personality that you must experience, challenge, and heal in order to create authentic power while you help bring to another awareness of the frightened parts of her personality that she must experience, challenge, and heal.

Did you review the Spiritual Partnership Guidelines before you began? Are you following them (experimenting with them) while you are supporting? The Spiritual Partnership Guidelines remind you of fundamentals and help you apply them to yourself as well as to the one you are supporting. For example, did you consult your intuition? Is your intention clear? (If your intention is not to support another, you are pursuing external power.) Are your observations and questions coming from the healthiest parts of your personality? Are you saying the things, when appropriate, that you fear might destroy your spiritual partnership? Are you in integrity?

When the person you are supporting reacts (for example, becomes angry, impatient, irritable, suspicious, or hostile) and a frightened part of your personality reacts to her reaction (for example, withdraws emotionally, defends, or meets anger with anger, impatience with impatience, or hostility with hostility), you enter a struggle for external power. A frightened part of your personality chose to participate, but only you can choose to end your participation.

The frightened part of your personality that is attracted to the struggle intends to win. It is convinced that its cause is just, that the other is at fault, or incorrect, or inferior. In other words, it is threatened and pursues external power. Only you can challenge this part of your personality. When you step out of a power struggle, even while that part of your personality refuses, you challenge that part. It continues to feel painful sensations, think angry thoughts, and intend to vanquish its opponent, and you continue to experience these things, but instead of acting on them you cease to participate in the struggle. You remain silent if necessary (with the intention to create authentic power), leave the room if necessary (with the intention to create authentic power), or listen as attentively as you can at the moment (with the intention to create authentic power). Any other intention for remaining silent, leaving, or listening is the pursuit of external power.

Supporting another in creating authentic power requires you to draw upon your intuition, courage, and compassion. Can you do that when you are upset, jealous, frustrated, or impatient? It requires love instead of fear, and challenging fear when love is not present. Can you challenge the frightened parts of your personality when the one you support will not challenge hers? It demands the conscious intention to support the creation of authentic power. Can you include yourself in that intention?

The purpose of spiritual partnerships is spiritual growth, and your participation in them supports you in every way to grow spiritually.

32

Spiritual Partnership in Action 2

Opportunities to create authentic power and spiritual partnerships are everywhere. Whenever you discover that a frightened part of your personality is active and whenever you see that a frightened part of another personality is active, or you think that one might be, you have an opportunity to create authentic power and, possibly, a spiritual partnership. For example, when someone complains to you (or about you), gossips, criticizes himself or others, creates an "us" and "them" orientation, or looks to you for approval, a frightened part of his personality is active. If he feels superior or inferior, a frightened part of his personality is active. When an individual is angry, anxious, resentful, jealous, depressed, or manic, a frightened part of his personality is active. When he cannot stop drinking alcohol, using drugs, smoking, gambling, watching pornography, having sex, or shopping, a frightened part of his personality is active. Whenever you notice obsessive thinking (such as savior searching, vengeful thoughts, etc.), compulsive activity (such as workaholism, perfectionism, etc.), or addictive behavior (such as alcoholism, overeating, etc.), a frightened part of a personality is active.

Wherever you go, wherever you look, whomever you encounter, you will see individuals with frightened parts of their personalities active. Every smile with a second agenda (for example, to put you at ease, seduce you, or sell you) reveals a frightened part of a personality. So also does every snarl, scowl, and frown. All of these are attempts to manipulate and control, and all of them are painful (for the manipulator). Anger, for example, is the pursuit of external power, and it is painful to experience. So also are jealousy, vengefulness, resentment, superiority, and inferiority.

Every painful emotion is a pursuit of external power. Five-sensory individuals think that painful emotions are caused by circumstances such as physical or psychological traumas, hormonal imbalances, or nutritional deficiencies and that the only remedies are physiological or environmental. They mistake correlates for causes. Every emotional experience has physiological, neurological, and environmental correlates, but these correlates do not cause the experience. They accompany it. Multisensory individuals see the pain of powerlessness beneath every psychological and psychiatric dysfunction, and creating authentic power as the remedy.

Understanding and developing emotional awareness transforms every painful emotion into a reminder that a frightened part of your personality is active and available to be challenged. In other words, the purpose of emotional pain is to help you grow spiritually. It brings your attention to parts of your personality that you need to heal in order to move into your full potential.

Multisensory humans do not refuse the benefits of therapy and pharmaceuticals if needed, just as individuals with physical damage do not refuse the benefits of emergency medicine, but they do not expect medicine or therapy to create an authentically powerful life for them. Eventually the torch must pass from dependence upon external circumstances to create happiness to dependence upon emotional awareness, responsible choice, intuition, and trust in the Universe to create joy.*

Five-sensory individuals do not make the connection be-

---

* Transiting from dependence on external circumstances in order to feel worthy and secure to creating authentic power also heals addictions (because addictions are the strongest frightened parts of the personality). The "Addiction" chapter in *The Seat of the Soul* (Gary Zukav, Simon & Schuster, 1989) leads you through the process of healing an addiction step-by-step. It uses sexual addiction as an example, but creating authentic power heals all addictions.

tween their painful emotions and their need to rearrange external circumstances. "I would do anything to be out of my pain," they think, but they are not willing to consider the possibility that the cause of it is inside them. "I hurt because I cannot have something that I want" (such as the return of a divorced spouse, a deceased loved one alive again, the success of a failed business, and so on), they explain, but they do not learn from their painful experiences. If they suddenly obtained what they cannot have (for example, the divorced spouse returns, the loved one does not die, the failing business succeeds), their pain would disappear. If they were looking, they would see that needing the world to be different caused their pain. ("There is suffering" and "Desire is the cause of suffering" are the Buddha's first two Noble Truths.)

Five-sensory humans attempt to momentarily avoid the pain of powerlessness by rearranging the world. They sympathize, empathize, comfort, and help friends change the circumstances that appear to cause their emotional pain, and they expect help in return when they need it. They pursue external power. Multisensory humans who are creating authentic power permanently heal the pain of powerlessness. They challenge and heal frightened parts of their personalities and cultivate loving parts of their personalities. They use the Spiritual Partnership Guidelines. Following are some examples of differences between the support that friends give to friends and the support that spiritual partners give to spiritual partners. Notice which kind of support you usually give.

SITUATION: An executive has been laid off, jobs are difficult to find, and his family depends upon him. His severance pay is gone, his unemployment insurance is running out, and although he has sent his résumé to many employers, he still has no job. He has never been without a job before or imagined that he would be.

FRIEND (fellow executive): You can find a job. Look where unemployment is low. Find out where venture capitalists are investing—in energy, biotech, green, etc.—and go there. Create a tour of several cities and visit four or five companies in each. Present yourself in person. Don't go through the human resources department. I always listen when someone is brave enough to put himself in my office uninvited. Call me when you need to. I'll be there for you when you want to kick some ideas around.

SPIRITUAL PARTNER: What are you feeling? What are the sensations in your body? Do you think these are sensations of loving parts of your personality or frightened parts of your personality? Have you felt sensations like these in other situations? What thoughts are you thinking? Do you think these are the thoughts of a loving part of your personality or a frightened part? Have you noticed thoughts like these at other times in your life? What is your intention in talking with me (for example, to complain, justify, vent anger or frustration, judge others, judge "the system," challenge frightened parts of your personality)? Is this the intention of a loving part of your personality or a frightened part? This is an opportunity for you to challenge frightened parts of your personality that are very painful and that existed before you were hired for your first job. Do you want to heal them?

Frightened parts of your personality are active, and this circumstance gives you an opportunity to experience, challenge, and heal them. If you don't, they will become active again and you will have another opportunity, but why not challenge them now? The more you do, the more effective (and fulfilled) you will be in finding a new job and everything else.

I will help you find a job, but this opportunity is greater than finding a job.

SITUATION: A professional man learns that his wife wants to divorce. They have two children. Their relationship has been strained, but he did not expect this. He cannot sleep, his work is suffering, and so is he. He calls a friend.

FRIEND: Meet me at the bar and we'll talk about this over drinks. . . . (*At the bar*) Scotch for me. What will you have? I know this is difficult, but it's not the end of the world. When my first wife left me I thought I would die, but it turned out to be the best thing. It was tough on the children, but they adjust. We all do. . . . *We'll have two more.* . . . It was hard at the office, but I managed. People can be supportive when you need them. You're a great guy, handsome, hardworking, successful. Any woman would love to get you. Just open to new possibilities. . . . *Give us another round.* . . . Have you noticed that my secretary has been eyeing you for months? I know she wants to meet you. She is a great person, beautiful, single. I could speak to her about getting together sometime—you, me, her, and my wife. What do you think about that? . . . *Give us another round.*

SPIRITUAL PARTNER: Meet me at the restaurant. . . . (*At the restaurant*) What's happening? What are you feeling in your chest? Have you felt that before in your life? That is because it is not coming from your wife's decision. It is coming from a part of your personality that existed before you met your wife. If you do not heal it, it will come again, no matter how many more women you find or marry. What thoughts are you having? Have you had thoughts like these before? They are experiences of this part of your personality, too. What is your intention for speaking now (to complain, be saved, use this experience to grow in healthy ways)?

Why waste this experience when you can use it to heal the inner sources of your terrible pain? This pain comes from frightened parts of your personality. You cannot heal these parts of your personality by blaming your wife, blaming yourself, or pitying yourself. You cannot heal them by distracting yourself with alcohol, sex, eating, work, sports, or anything else. Instead you can experience these painful parts of your personality as fully as you can, and *while you are experiencing them,* deliberately choose a different intention than they would choose, do something constructive that they would not do. The more you challenge them while you are feeling them, the more they lose their ability to disrupt your life.

SITUATION: A four-year-old girl (our granddaughter) jubilantly rides her bicycle without training wheels for the first time. "Look at me! Look at me!" she shouts in joy to her admiring father, grandmother (Linda), and me. Her six-year-old sister withdraws by herself to a grassy spot, sits motionlessly, and stares at her feet.

FRIEND (grandmother who doesn't use the Spiritual Partnership Guidelines): What's wrong, Honey?

GIRL: My sister is getting all the attention.

FRIEND: Don't worry. Daddy loves you very much. He is just cheering your sister on. You have a prettier bicycle than your sister anyway. You know that, don't you? Would you like to get an ice-cream cone, just you and me? I know a special place I bet you haven't been to!

SPIRITUAL PARTNER (Linda): What is happening with you, Honey?

GIRL: My sister is getting all the attention.

SPIRITUAL PARTNER: That doesn't feel good, does it? What do you feel? Do you feel anything in your chest? That doesn't feel good, does it? Do you feel anything in your stomach? That doesn't feel good, either, does it? Do you want to keep feeling these things? You can stay here and continue to feel these things, or you could try an experiment. You could go over to your sister and congratulate her for riding her bicycle without training wheels. Would you like to do that?

GIRL: Congratulations. You really looked good. (Sister beams.)

SPIRITUAL PARTNER: How do you feel now?

GIRL: I feel better! It worked!

SPIRITUAL PARTNER: You can experiment by yourself the next time you are not feeling good.

There are countless examples of friends supporting friends around you. How many examples of spiritual partners supporting spiritual partners are there? How many would you like to see? You can create examples for your friends as well as your spiritual partners by using the Spiritual Partnership Guidelines wherever you are, whatever you are doing. There is no time that is not appropriate for commitment to growing spiritually, courage to experience what you are feeling, compassion for yourself and others, conscious communications and actions, integrity, emotional awareness, responsible choices, intuition, and trust in the Universe. When these are absent, your interactions take you further along the horizontal path (circumstances change but you do not), and you continue to create the same experiences with the same frightened parts of your personality. When they are present, you take the vertical path (you change), frightened parts of your personality create fewer and fewer destructive consequences for you, and loving parts of your personality create more and more constructive consequences.

33

Soul Summary

SPIRITUAL PARTNERSHIPS—HOW

- The Spiritual Partnership Guidelines help you create authentic power and spiritual partnership in every situation.
- Commitment, courage, compassion, and conscious communications and actions are required to create authentic power and spiritual partnerships.
- The Spiritual Partnership Guidelines help you develop each step-by-step.
- Creating spiritual partnerships requires creating authentic power.
- When you follow the Spiritual Partnership Guidelines you create authentic power no matter what others do.
- The Spiritual Partnership Guidelines are evolving.
- Creating authentic power enables you to participate in the evolution of the Spiritual Partnership Guidelines.
- You must follow the Spiritual Partnership Guidelines (not just talk about them or think about them) to create authentic power and spiritual partnerships.

You can create a spiritual partnership with anyone who is committed to becoming more aware, responsible, and healthy—to decreasing fear in her life and increasing love. Race, religion, culture, sex, nationality, and economic circumstance are not barriers. Frightened parts of your personality are barriers, and as you challenge and heal them, they influence you less and less.

No list is long enough to include the *Who* you can create spiritual partnerships with, but a few of the most common and important collectives that all of us interact with are included in the following section. How many more can you think of? Include them, too.

WHO

34

Families

No relationships offer more possibilities for spiritual growth than relationships between children and parents. They are the most intense and far-reaching relationships, the most substantive, and the most impactful. They are also far more complex, deep, and powerful than they appear to five-sensory perception.

Interactions between souls that are parents and souls that are children begin prior to birth and continue after death. For example, when the soul of a child leaves the Earth school before the souls of its parents (for example, the child dies at birth or is killed in an accident or as a soldier), interactions between them continue.

Whether your family experiences were gentle or brutal, interactions between you, your parents, and your siblings, if you have any, serve the healing of all involved. In one family a mother may be dominating (frightened) and in another meek and submissive (frightened); in one family the father may be able to show his love only through his financial support of the family (frightened) and in another be an abusive alcoholic (frightened). No family is without pain, because no family members are without frightened parts of the personality.

The influence of parents on children and of children on parents and the love between them cannot be overestimated. That love is the bond that brings souls into a family, predates the personalities involved, and continues after they leave the Earth school. Even in families where a parent is so brutal and disconnected (frightened) that his or her departure is a relief rather than a sorrow, there remains a longing to continue the relationship. This is not merely because of dependence (fear). It is an experience of the love that connects each family member and pervades his or her experiences, no matter how painful and brutal they may be.

When a child is adopted, even at birth, she enters into another family dynamic that also serves her spiritual growth, but the influence of her birth family continues to affect her and be felt. The parents will never forget their child although they may believe that they have. The connection between them cannot be broken, and eventually one will begin to think of the other. "Does he think of me? Would he want to see me again? Is she a professor? A housewife? Lost in drugs? (Oh, I hope not.) What does my daughter look like? What kind of a person is my mother? (I think I know!)" These are the kinds of thoughts that emerge and reemerge in separated parents and children, no matter how long they have been apart. They are experiences of the indestructible bond between them that continues even as new circumstances unfold and, when new families are involved, interweave with those new family experiences.

During my last year in college, a girl that I was seeing became pregnant. Although we were confused and frightened, we both knew that we were not able to raise a child. Our daughter was born while I was in the army, and she was adopted at birth. For several years I did not think about her. In fact, I discovered later that my reason for enlisting in the army was to avoid facing the very things that frightened me the most. Eventually I began to wonder where she was, what she was doing, and if she was well and happy. I continued to wonder about her for years. "My daughter is thirteen this year," I would think. "My daughter is nineteen this year." "This year she is twenty-three." "What is she doing now?" "Is she happy?" When *The Dancing Wu Li Masters* was published I fantasized that she might recognize my name and contact me. More years passed. I found her mother. She also did not know anything about our daughter except the name of the hospital where she was born. Laws separating birth parents from their adopted children were omnipresent and effective at that time. At last I found a kind person who helped reconnect biological parents with their children. I gave her the little information I had, and months later she called to tell me that she had located my daughter.

I couldn't move or breathe. I could barely answer her. I was filled with fear of the information I had sought so long. I wrote down the address and phone number she gave me, thanked her, and remained motionless at my desk. I thought I would be thrilled, but I was terrified. I couldn't pick up the telephone again. I looked at the information in my hand again and again for weeks, thinking of what I would do with it. Should I call? What if she didn't want to see me? What if she was angry—how could she not be? Worst of all, what if she wouldn't talk to me? What if I would never know if my daughter was happy, if she had been treated well, if she was married? That thought suddenly jolted me—What if she has children! In retrospect it seems impossible that it had not occurred to me before, but the possibility that my daughter had children filled me with wonder—and then with fear that I might not be able to see them.

I spent weeks gathering my courage and preparing to call her. I imagined every reaction that she might have—rage, fear, curiosity, acceptance. Would she angrily hang up, disdain me, or be relieved? When I called she was startled, but she spoke with me at once, and continued to speak with me. She told me of her life and her family (she had a daughter!). As she spoke, I felt an experience beyond any joy I had felt. It seemed to me that my daughter *wanted to share herself* with me! Whatever she was feeling, I was filled with awe and gratitude. We made plans to speak again and said good-bye. I could not move or think. Emotions that I could not recognize or distinguish at the time filled me, and I loved them all. They were so deep and meaningful, so rich and comforting. My daughter was well! My daughter was well! My daughter was loved!

I cried and laughed at these wondrous things. Then fear returned. Would she speak with me again? What if she changed her mind? Each new thought of fear plunged me into pain again, and so began the recommencement of one of the most meaningful stories of my life, one that I had sought to push away from my thoughts and ignore as though it had not happened. It had happened, it was happening, and now, twenty-seven years later, I stepped back into it as consciously as I could. It is still happening, and every year my gratitude for the Universe, for my life, and for my daughter deepens. I am still amazed that someone as angry and uncaring as I had been could feel such strong and loving emotions about my daughter given up for adoption so many years ago.

Our story is not unlike millions of others—of the pain of an abortion that reemerges years later with staggering intensity, or never left; the excruciating longing for a child given away; or the prolonged pain of marrying out of fear in order to provide a child a home. Parents and children are affected by one another not only in these dramatic ways. As we become multisensory we see that all of our interactions with our parents and our children are substantive and deep. Frightened parts of the personalities of our parents affect us, and frightened parts of our personalities affect our children.

Parents fear their children as well as love them. Every father needs to be admired by his son, to be worthy of his respect, wonders if he will be, and fears that he will not. Every mother needs to be loved by her daughter, to model goodness and health, wonders if she will be, and fears in her hidden places (frightened parts of her personality) that she will not. The frightened parts of the personality of every parent need the approval of his or her child or children. In no other kind of relationship are you challenged more often and deeply, and offered opportunities to create authentic power more frequently and persistently, than in your family.

Your family is your "homeroom" in the Earth school. All that you learn in your other classrooms relate to or weave back into your experiences with your family. Throughout your journey through the Earth school your interactions with your family shape and pervade your experiences. You might see in yourself, for example, your father's temper, disdain, gentleness, or inferiority, or your mother's need to control or please, her inferiority or her superiority. Frightened parts of their personalities appear as parts of your own. For example, I once heard my father's voice coming from my mouth with exactly the intonation that I disliked intensely in him. I wanted to rip it out of me, but I didn't know how. The more frightened I became, the more like my father I sounded. Since I didn't understand at the time what a "frightened part of the personality" is or how to recognize it, I didn't know how to challenge it. I thought it was "the way I am," the unchangeable ground of my being that destined me to be like my father in the same way that genes and chromosomes destined me to have his physical characteristics, and I continued to hear and abhor my father's voice in my own.

The physical characteristics that children acquire from their parents—a smile or way of laughing, body shape, artistic or musical ability, intellectual agility—and that their parents acquired in turn from their parents, and so on, are transmitted genetically. The frightened parts of a personality have a deeper origin than genes, chromosomes, or environment. They are aspects of the soul that the soul desires to heal through the choices of its personality. Their origin is not physical. In other words, you did not inherit them from your parents, and interactions with your parents did not create them. You entered the Earth school with them, and interactions with your family activated (and activate) them. Although you become irritable, withdrawn, rebellious, judgmental, terrified, and enraged by members of your family, these same experiences will torment you again and again until you heal the frightened parts of your personality that generate them. That is the creation of authentic power.

Your struggles and the struggles of your parents interlock. The strengths that you need to develop in order to interact lovingly with your parents are the same strengths that you need to develop in order to move into your full potential and to give the gifts that you were born to give. You can move away from your family, but you cannot move away from the frightened parts of your personality. You can refuse to speak with your family, but the frightened parts of your personality will continue to speak with you. You cannot outrun them, hide from them, or avoid them. Interactions with your family, even if your parents are deceased or you have not met them, are the "ground zero" of these experiences.

From the five-sensory perspective, random events bring personalities together as parents, and random combinations of chromosomes and genes determine the characteristics of their children. From a multisensory perspective, souls that agree to become parents if certain conditions come into being and souls that agree to become their children if certain conditions come into being agree prior to incarnation to support one another in the Earth school to grow spiritually. In other words, your parents and you, and you and your children, are perfect for one another.

The history of a family affects its members, and their interactions affect future members. This is generational karma. In biblical terms, the sins of the parent are visited upon the child. In the vocabulary of authentic power, the unhealed frightened parts of a personality are experienced by descendents of that personality until they are challenged and healed. That changes the generational karma of the family. Collectives such as race, culture, and nation as well as families create karma. The karma of each is an energetic lineage, or inheritance, just as physical characteristics that are passed from generation to generation in a family are a genetic lineage.

From the five-sensory perspective, healing a frightened part of your personality heals only you. From the multisensory perspective, it changes the generational karma of your family. Your children do not inherit that frightened part of your personality from you, and their children do not inherit it from them. From a five-sensory perspective, only the future can be changed. From a multisensory perspective, previous generations of a family are healed when a family member heals a frightened part of his or her personality, all the way back to the origin of that part in the family. In other words, creating authentic power affects your family's past as well as its future.

The soul has many personalities, all exist simultaneously, and each has a lineage. Your lineage may be black, white, yellow, brown, or red; male or female; Muslim, Christian, or Hindu; French, Australian, or Thai, but you are much more than that. Each of us can say, "I have been a male. I have been a female. I have been a mother and I have been a father." Some can say, "I have been Chinese and I have been Egyptian." Others can say, "I have been a Mongolian warrior on the steppes and I have been a slave." Still others can say, "I have been a Catholic priest and I have been a Druid." This expanded perception is beyond the capabilities of the five senses, but it is part of multisensory perception.

The five-sensory perception of the family as the unique, defining, and sole origin of the personality is being replaced by the multisensory perception of the family as a vehicle chosen by souls to assist one another in spiritual development, repeatedly, in many times and in many places. When you create a spiritual partnership in your family, you access a healing potential that is far greater than it appears.

35
Friends

Friendships are as different from spiritual partnerships as aquatic creatures are from humans who walk upright on the Earth. In the evolution of physical form, aquatic life from its simplest to its most complex forms culminated in organisms capable of temporarily leaving the oceans (amphibians). Then came air-breathing creatures completely adapted to living and thriving on the surface of the Earth. No one with knowledge of the amazing record of evolution that has been preserved in fossils, and the curiosity and intelligence to read it, doubts that water-breathing forms of Life preceded air-breathing forms of Life on the Earth. Water-based and land-based organisms are entirely different, sharing only the Life that both express. Anyone who has inhaled water in a pool or the ocean knows that breathing water does not serve human evolution.

Friendship and spiritual partnership are also entirely different, sharing only the need for relationship that both express. Just as water-based organisms served the evolution of Life on the Earth prior to the appearance of land-based organisms, friendships served the evolution of humanity prior to the appearance of multisensory perception. Multisensory individuals do not choke on friendships as air-breathing forms of Life choke on water, but as multisensory humans become accustomed to their expanded perception of themselves and others as more than bodies and minds with goals beyond survival and comfort, they discover that friendships do not satisfy them as much as they once did, sometimes even their closest friendships.

Multisensory individuals do not eschew friendships or friends. They instead are attracted to interactions that are not part of friendships and that, in fact, threaten friendships. Friendships and spiritual partnerships are both vehicles for reaching out in love and caring for others, but friendships are designed to serve the needs of five-sensory individuals, and spiritual partnerships are designed to fulfill the needs of multisensory individuals. Five-sensory individuals need to pursue external power and survive in order to evolve, and multisensory individuals need to create authentic power and grow spiritually in order to evolve. Pursuing external power is as counterproductive for multisensory humans as attempting to breathe underwater (it is lethal), and alignment of the personality with the soul is as meaningless to five-sensory humans as lungs would be to aquatic creatures, if they had intellects and could inquire about "lungs." "What are lungs for?" they would ask, and no fellow aquatic creature would be able to provide an answer. "What are spiritual partnerships for?" five-sensory individuals ask, and no fellow five-sensory individuals can provide an experientially meaningful answer.

As we transit from a five-sensory to a multisensory humanity, the new overlaps the old, friendships abound, spiritual partnerships are emerging—even though they are not always recognized or labeled as such—and both coexist. This can be confusing, especially when some friends awaken to a desire for more than friendships can offer and others do not. The foundation of their friendships begins to shift, and the structures resting on it become unstable. They continue to care for one another (best-case scenario), but they find fewer mutual interests. Spiritual partners discuss children, health, jobs, education, styles, and family challenges with one another as do friends, but they do it from a different perspective. They look for what they can learn about themselves in order to heal the frightened parts of their personalities and cultivate the loving parts.

Friends look for what they can change or fix for others in order to make others or themselves feel better. They do not understand that only frightened parts of the personality (not people or circumstances) can create pain in themselves and their friends. Therefore, they strive to satisfy the needs of frightened parts of one another's personalities. When a friend loses a job, for example, friends sympathize or empathize, listen to his distress, give him advice, and wish him well. Spiritual partners support him in experiencing what he is feeling, identifying frightened parts of his personality, and healing them. They help him clarify his intentions—for example, if he is blaming his boss for his misfortune instead of focusing on the painful physical sensations that he is feeling and responding to the frightened parts of his personality instead of reacting to them. They see the cause of their friend's upset and pain—a frightened part of his personality—and support him in healing it.

If a romance or marriage dissolves, friends agree about the villain and sympathize with the victim. They share stories of similar losses and lessons learned. They arrange distractions to keep their friend out of pain. Spiritual partners help her eradicate the pain by healing the frightened parts of her personality that cause it. In other words, friends focus on the experiences of frightened parts of the personality (I am lost, helpless, hopeless, lonely, and so on), and spiritual partners focus on how to heal those parts. Friends help one another change what activates the frightened parts of their personalities, and spiritual partners help one another change what is activated.

This is the difference between the pursuit of external power and the creation of authentic power. Pursuing external power requires changing your external circumstances. Creating authentic power requires changing your internal dynamics. These differences in perception, purpose, and method make the interactions of spiritual partners surprising and sometimes unwelcome by friends and nurturing and welcome by other spiritual partners and potential spiritual partners. When your intention is to heal a frightened part of your personality that blames others for a painful experience, for example, friends who agree with that part of your personality cannot help you. Frightened parts of their personalities join with yours. ("I would have done the same thing in your place." "How could he have done such a thing!" "She clearly has no scruples.") They do not hold the intention to heal the frightened parts of their personalities, and so they do not understand your intention to heal yours.

Friends try to help fix the situation, make it right instead of wrong, and if they cannot they assure you that it will work out better next time. Circumstances change, but the frightened parts of the personality work the same way each time they become active, and the pain they create is the same. Spiritual partners know this, but friends do not think about it. Friends are not aware of their internal experiences except when emotional pain forces itself into their consciousness, and so they cannot assist one another in exploring their internal experiences. On the contrary, they mask them with caretaking, fixing, advising, and sympathizing, and so their efforts to reach out in love become attempts to manipulate and control. For example, when a friend smiles instead of cries, they feel better. When a friend agrees instead of disagrees, they feel better. They feel better when a friend accepts their support instead of rejecting it.

The intention to pursue external power goes unnoticed because friends are not always interested in intentions. Spiritual partners pay close attention to their intentions. Friends help one another succeed because succeeding is important to them. Spiritual partners help one another heal frightened parts of their personalities and cultivate loving parts because that is important to them. Friends commit to maintaining friendships. Spiritual partners commit to growing spiritually. Friends expect the support of friends, and they are disappointed, hurt, or angry when they do not receive it. In other words, they attempt to change one another when frightened parts of their personalities become active. Spiritual partners intend to heal frightened parts of their personalities when they become active. This is another way of saying that friends perceive power as the ability to manipulate and control external circumstances, and spiritual partners perceive it as the ability to change their internal circumstances.

Friends strive to stay in their comfort zones (avoid experiencing frightened parts of their personalities). If a frightened part of your personality that procrastinates, for example, explodes in anger when someone mentions your procrastination, your friends quickly learn not to mention it to you. If you become morose or melancholy when you think of your mother who passed on, your friends do not discuss her with you or they sympathize with you. If you struggle with a need for alcohol, excessive food, nicotine, or shopping, your friends will not ask why these things are irresistible to you. In fact, they will participate in them with you and defend you and themselves if others inquire. Their goal is not to uncover the painful dynamics beneath their behaviors that are out of control. On the contrary, it is to keep those dynamics buried beneath distracting (obsessive, compulsive, and addictive) experiences and behaviors.

The price that friends—and everyone else—pay to remain in their comfort zones is uncontrollable destructive behaviors that erupt without warning or restraint into their lives—spiteful words, rageful deeds, acts of resentment and jealousy, power struggles, and more. Some cannot stop drinking, smoking, or masturbating. Some hunt incessantly for sex, others shop uncontrollably, others need to dominate those around them, and yet others need to please those around them. Some feel inferior and others feel superior. Some need to be the center of attention and others withdraw emotionally. Arguments with spouses and children recur.

Friends become former friends, gossip, and sometimes become vengeful. The flip from attraction to repulsion, "love" to disdain can happen very fast. Sometimes friends of many years cease to speak to one another, and even parents and children or siblings become estranged.

Spiritual partners travel beyond the boundaries of their comfort zones. They do not seek the temporary security and well-being of a frightened part of the personality that has acquired for the moment what it needs in order to feel safe and valuable. They seek the joy of loving without reservation. Beyond comfort lie the painful physical sensations of frightened parts of the personality, and there also lies the ability to replace them with blissful experiences of loving parts of the personality. Attachment to comfort is avoidance of discomfort. It closes the mind, barricades the heart, and confines the one who is attached to the company of those who also fear to experience discomfort. Fear creates the need to be with those who avoid exploring the frightened parts of their personalities, fear creates destructive behaviors and consequences, and fear prevents exploring their origins. Friendships were not designed to support individuals in exploring and healing the frightened parts of their personalities. That goal was not part of the evolution of five-sensory humanity.

Spiritual partnerships are designed precisely for that. Their purpose is to support equals in the creation of authentic power through the conscious use of their interactions. Spiritual partnerships require commitment, courage, compassion, and conscious communications and actions. Spiritual partners care for one another. Their bond is as deep as the bond between friends, but it serves a significantly different goal—evolution through spiritual growth instead of survival, the creation of authentic power instead of external power.

Transforming friendships into spiritual partnerships does not require changing others (that is the pursuit of external power). It requires changing you. All that is needed to create the potential for a spiritual partnership is commitment to creating authentic power and following the Spiritual Partnership Guidelines. The Spiritual Partnership Guidelines show you how to change yourself, not others. What difference does it make what others are doing when your intention is to learn about yourself from your interactions with them—to notice your emotions, thoughts, and intentions? When your intention is to practice integrity at all times, what difference does it make what others intend? When you intend to take responsibility for your experiences instead of blaming, what difference does it make if others blame? When you respond to frightened parts of your personality instead of react, you attract individuals who do the same. When a flower blooms, bees find it.

Spiritual partnerships grow as naturally as sprouts grow from seeds. Creating authentic power plants the seeds. You cannot convert, persuade, or convince others to become spiritual partners, but you can create authentic power, model it in the process, and the Law of Attraction will work for you.

Creating spiritual partnerships requires willingness to experiment with speaking and acting in different ways than you have before. Not all of your friends will be attracted to taking responsibility for their experiences, saying what is difficult to say when it is appropriate, becoming aware of their interior experiences, choosing their intentions consciously, being vulnerable, and using their experiences with you to grow spiritually. You will find your relationships with them becoming less interesting. Others will respond with an interest in making your friendships more substantive and meaningful, and those are potential spiritual partners.

Creating a spiritual partnership is as natural as finding a "friend," except that this friend is interested in changing herself for the better instead of holding others responsible for why she is not changing, for taking responsibility for her experiences instead of blaming them on parents, peers, her boss, or her workload, and giving the gifts that she was born to give. The commitment to self-exploration and self-knowledge, conscious and responsible creation, consulting intuition, and experimenting with the Universe in the intimate context of everyday interactions produces a new and more meaningful type of relationship that goes beyond what friends can offer one another—partnership between equals for the purpose of spiritual growth.

You will not attempt to mollify, pacify, or placate this new kind of "friend," and she will not want you to. A spiritual partner does not want frightened parts of his personality to be mollified, pacified, or placated, especially when he is reactive. That is when he is most intent on experiencing them and challenging them, for example, when he is in a power struggle, angered by a perceived rudeness, jealous, or feeling depressed. When a participant at one of the events in our three-year program received news before a session that her brother had committed suicide, she stood waiting for Linda at the entrance to the meeting room, trembling. She did not want to be consoled, pitied, uplifted, or advised. She wanted a spiritual partner who understood the internal origin of her pain and her need not to be fixed. She wanted to feel the full power of a frightened part of her personality in order to challenge and heal it. Linda took her into her arms, and they stood silently while she felt her emotions and drew upon the support of Linda and the spiritual partners around her. The moment was not sentimental or sorrowful. It was powerful.

Spiritual partners are tender, caring, direct, and open. They love one another enough to brave the reactions of frightened parts of one another's personalities in order to create authentic power and support one another in creating authentic power. Laughter and tears flow easily when no fears hold them back. The more you become able to experience and challenge your reactions, in all their pain and power, the more you become able to support your spiritual partners in creating authentic power and be supported by them, and the more you fill with compassion for others—those who are friends and those who are not, those who are kind and those who are cruel, those who create authentic power and those who yet pursue external power.

36

Coworkers

The military, religion, and commerce are sibling organizations. They are each highly structured, coordinated, and effective pursuits of external power. Only their dogmas, uniforms, and methods differ. All are global, ignore the boundaries of cultures, nations, and individuals, and strive for dominance. They are proactive, competitive, and expansive in nature, obliterating if possible all values except their own and suppressing opposing values if not. Highly homogenous, they do not allow diversity except where necessary and when it serves their objectives. They aggressively impose themselves to the best of their ability.

They assimilate or eliminate adversaries. Beneath exterior differences lies the same intention—to manipulate and control through force of arms, ideas, or money. No resources are withheld. All weapons are brought to bear continually—cannons, canons, and currency—with the sole goal of dominating nations, cultures, and competitors. Contentment is not a part of military, religious, or commercial organizations. Soldiers train to wage war and impatiently wait for opportunities in times of peace. Priests, monks, and missionaries spread their ideas continually, ceaselessly competing with conflicting ideologies. Commercial success demands ever-expanding market share and endlessly increasing profits for investors.

All three present themselves in the most appealing way possible while pursuing objectives that are not always appealing. Military organizations appeal to national pride and ideology. Currently, for example, they present themselves as defenders of nationhood, democracy, and freedom, yet few military organizations remain defensive when offense is possible. From warring tribes to multimillion-person armies, military organizations have raided neighbors and conquered nations, stolen horses and oil reserves, forced individuals into slavery or destitution, and in countless ways imposed themselves by force. Not every soldier is aggressive and brutal, but the function and purpose of every military organization is.

No religion feeds the hungry or cares for the poor without a second agenda to proselytize. Its good deeds come with a price ("believe as we believe"). The righteous are saved, infidels are punished, heretics are killed, heresy is eradicated, and opposing beliefs are eliminated, displaced, or assimilated. Not all religious individuals (such as Mother Teresa) care for the needy in order to convert nonbelievers, but all religious organizations do.

No business pursues a greater goal than net income. Slogans such as Progress Is Our Most Important Product and Working Together for a Green World are disconnected from ever-perfected practices to produce maximal profit. Profit Is Our Most Important Product is the anthem of every corporation—automotive, telecom, steel, software, and more—but proclaimed by none except banks. The lack of connection between sound-bite logos and the environmental pollution, destruction of forests, poisoning of towns, scarring of mountains, fouling of the atmosphere, and extinction of species that commercial organizations create results from the pursuit of external power. Like chameleons changing colors to blend into their surroundings, businesses become "community oriented," then "environmentally friendly," then "energy efficient," to project contemporary images of social sensitivity and responsibility that mask the ultimate, only, and unyielding objective of all corporate endeavors—to maximize shareholder profits and executive bonuses.

The values, methods, and objectives of these organizations shape individuals within them. Soldiers, religious professionals, and businesspeople recognize one another in or out of uniform. Each of these organizations—military, religious, and commercial—crushes or discourages individuality, constrains original thinking, and confines creativity to acceptable channels. All members of the military fear individuals with higher rank and failure to perform as required. Congregants fear ceaseless suffering or lack of enlightenment. Employees fear coworkers with more ability to manipulate and control, and executives fear the failure of their business to profit. In short, each of these organizations is built upon the perception of power as external and relentlessly pursues it.

The measure of commercial activity is called an *economy*. No one has ever seen an economy. There are local, national, international, and global economies, all of them yet to be photographed. They differ in scale (the number of commercial activities they measure), but they are essentially the same. They could not exist without commercial endeavors (businesses), and so they reflect the businesses that they measure. The total value of the goods and services created in a nation measures the activity of all the businesses in the nation. Since many commercial organizations do business in several countries on different continents, through different suborganizations and ownership structures, in order to maximize profits (and bonuses) and reduce taxes, the global economy has become more important in the last century. It is very important today because it affects businesses everywhere, even those that are not international, not corporations, and not large.

An economy is a picture of commercial activity painted in broad strokes. While some businesses in an economy may grow and others fail, the economy does not describe these things. It shows an overall picture that includes all of these activities, large and small, successful (profitable) and not. When an economy grows (the value of the goods and services produced increases), that is considered good (because more businesses profit, more and bigger bonuses are paid, and shareholders get larger returns from their investments). The opposite happens when an economy does not grow or contracts. That is considered bad. Therefore, the more that businesses produce and sell, the better the economy is said to be.

An economy does not take into account the effects of the commercial activities in it on, for example, youth, the elderly, communities that host businesses, the well-being of employees, care of pregnant women, or education for young people. It does not take into account their effects on the environment, quality of life, health, global warming, or the well-being of the Earth, humanity, and other forms of Life. It measures only monetary value (money). It also reflects the pursuit of external power that generates five-sensory businesses.

This is the reflection: When something (for example, apples) is not easily available (supply) and many people want it (demand), the price increases, and the reverse. Every economy assumes a shared intention of the individuals involved in commercial activities to maximize self-benefit (profit) at all costs (to others). These assumptions are not made by economies since economies are not real things. They are made by people who study economies, and they accurately describe the continual pursuit of five-sensory individuals to manipulate and control (and take advantage of) circumstances in order to make themselves feel safe and valuable.

In short, commercial organizations (businesses) are pursuits of external power embedded in a statistical entity (economy) that assumes this pursuit. Not all individuals in commercial activities act in their own self-interest all of the time, but all commercial organizations do.

At jobsites, in offices, stores, and fields, workers participate in five-sensory endeavors that reflect the requirements of a five-sensory species that is evolving through the pursuit of external power. The perception of power as the ability to manipulate and control is now counterproductive, but commercial organizations that are built upon it and economies that reflect it continue to exist. Like cars that have run out of gas and yet continue to roll down the freeway, sometimes for a long distance if they were traveling fast when their fuel disappeared, commercial organizations and the economies that describe their activities have run out of fuel, no more is available, and none will be. All are pursuits of external power, and external power now prevents our evolution.

No matter how understanding your boss, congenial your coworkers, and constructive the products or services that your company provides, the enterprise itself is the pursuit of external power, and the participation of five-sensory individuals within it serves the toxic pursuit of external power. No matter how many benefits or lack of them employees receive, the bottom line of every corporation is net revenue, and all intelligence, creativity, and resources available are continually directed toward maximizing it (and bonuses). This occurs whether or not employees have invested in the company stock or are eligible for bonuses; whether they are executives, managers, clerks, or janitors; whether customers of the enterprise are individuals or other companies. Quality of service and excellence of product have no value to the enterprise apart from increasing its net revenue. Employees also have no value to the enterprise apart from increasing its net revenue.

This is the context in which coworkers interact. It appears to be shockingly disconnected from ourselves, a grotesque portrait of an alien consciousness, but is it? We reel at the monstrosity before us and around us and wonder what our relationship with it could be. Like spectators at a movie that we did not expect to see, we are surprised and confused. We blame the actors for this dismal experience, but we do not know how to leave the theater. We blame the producers, director, and screenwriter; then we blame the cinematographer, makeup artists, and grips on the set. Still the movie plays on, and we continue to be absorbed in it without thinking about where we are (in a theater).

Circumstances recur. Coworkers gossip, seek allies against common threats, plot their advancement, are terrified by their managers, fear losing their jobs, and so on. Some behaviors of frightened parts of a personality are rewarded, such as workaholism and perfectionism ("detail oriented"), and others are punished, such as procrastination. A product is "rolled out," "public relations" begin, shareholders demand more, executives strive to provide it, and the security of everyone in the enterprise depends upon its success or failure.

The workplace is analogous to a theater. Employers are analogous to producers, managers are analogous to directors, supervisors are analogous to cinematographers, and fellow employees are analogous to actors. You are analogous to a viewer, totally absorbed in the movie, but your role is not as passive as it appears. *Your intentions appear on the big screen.* This goes unnoticed while you focus on the movie, but when you focus on your internal dynamics (frightened and loving parts of your personality), it becomes undeniable.

Frightened parts of your personality strive to obtain the most for the least (for example, shop for the best price). Obtaining the most for the least (maximal profit for minimal expense) is integral to the movie. Frightened parts of your personality seek advantage. Creating advantage (for example, outmaneuvering competitors) is central to the movie. Frightened parts of your personality fear not having enough. Fear of not having enough (for example, market share) is the theme of the movie. Once you recognize the intentions of the frightened parts of your personality, you cannot avoid recognizing them on the screen.

The shocking movie is not a creation of morally deformed individuals who create apart from you, profit apart from you, exploit apart from you, and seek value and security through the pursuit of external power apart from you. It reflects the intentions of frightened parts of *your* personality. They fuel the frightened parts of other personalities who appear to create and maintain this destructive system, but those individuals are not separate from you. They are your proxy creators.

The movie (workplace) that holds your attention captive is a micro-experience of the pursuit of external power that appears globally through the activities of international corporations, locally through the activities of businesses close to home, and intimately through the painful experiences that frightened parts of your personality create. It brings to the screen the needs and deeds of a five-sensory humanity that evolved through surviving. The needs and deeds of a multisensory humanity that evolves through growing spiritually require a different movie (kind of workplace). You create it when you create authentic power.

The old movie activates emotions in you, but each time you respond instead of react you change it. Whether you are promoted, demoted, "laid off," given a bonus, or told to stay home for a day (without pay), you change when you choose your words and actions consciously instead of unconsciously, and so does the movie. Your boss and colleagues may or may not notice the changes, but you do. The movie begins to lose its grip on you, and you become capable of experimenting within it.

Changing the movie does not require changing others (for example, your employer, manager, coworkers, and shareholders if there are any). It requires changing you. You change yourself when you use the Spiritual Partnership Guidelines, and the changes that you make in yourself change the movie. Your experiences with coworkers change. Each time you challenge a frightened part of your personality or cultivate a loving part you contribute differently to the collective consciousness, and the movie changes.

If a coworker begins to gossip, for example, and you use the Spiritual Partnership Guidelines instead of gossiping with her, the movie changes. When an abusive employer or vindictive coworker activates a frightened part of your personality and you challenge it instead of indulging it, the movie changes. When you see an employer or coworker as a soul who sometimes has frightened parts of his or her personality active instead of judging him or her, the movie changes. Each time you invoke healing—respond with emotional awareness and choose responsibly while a frightened part of your personality demands otherwise—the movie changes.

Five-sensory humans cannot see these changes because they can see only circumstances and other individuals. Multisensory humans see the movie change each time they draw power from a choice instead of lose power, each time they gain mastery in their lives that they did not have before. Instead of collapsing under the fear of the collective consciousness, they use it to create authentic power by challenging their own experiences of fear. They transform the collective consciousness through the force of their own consciousness. They challenge frightened parts of their personalities when the collective fear appears unchallengeable. They change the movie each time they create harmony instead of discord, share instead of hoard, cooperate instead of compete, and revere Life instead of exploit life.

A five-sensory human sees the fear-based nature of commerce as an unchangeable given in the human experience. A multisensory human recognizes it as a reflection of her internal dynamics. She knows that it cannot be changed without changing herself and that changing her internal dynamics is her responsibility. She welcomes her experiences at work, including her painful experiences, as opportunities to create authentic power and spiritual partnerships, and to participate in the transformation of commerce from a collective dynamic that fills the needs of frightened parts of the personality into a dynamic that brings the values of the soul into the Earth school.

37

Couples

Relationships between individuals who bond as couples are being transformed dramatically by the shift from old-type five-sensory relationships to new-type multisensory relationships. Their importance as the wellspring of human progeny is being replaced by their importance as intimate vehicles for creating authentic power. The birth of children enriches this dynamic and adds to its complexity. For example, the responsibilities of five-sensory parents to five-sensory children do not include the spiritual development of their children, not to be confused with religious education. From the five-sensory perspective, nurturing and protecting children serves the evolution of humankind by increasing its numbers and insures able-bodied support for aging parents. Five-sensory parents see themselves as personalities and their children as small, yet-to-develop versions of themselves.

Multisensory parents see themselves and their children as souls as well as personalities. They see spiritual development as the alignment of the personality with the soul. Exposing children to a religious tradition does not require transformation on the part of the parents. Creating authentic power and supporting children in creating authentic power does.

When five-sensory individuals bond, they see their relationship as a vehicle for bearing and raising children. They feel the pressure of parents and peers to become parents themselves. When multisensory individuals bond, they decide for themselves the functions that they will fill in their relationship (spiritual partners choose their own roles). Their choices may or may not include Father and Mother. The purpose of spiritual partnership between two individuals is spiritual growth whether or not they include parenthood in their shared journey. Their partnerships with each other and with their children, if they have any, are different from the relationships of five-sensory individuals, whose goals are survival and comfort.

Five-sensory couples are fulfilled by home and hearth, safety and comfort—just as their ancestors glowed with contentment around a fire after a successful hunt. Multisensory couples in pursuit of authentic power are fulfilled by challenging (and challenging again) frightened parts of their personalities that prevent them from sharing their love and giving the gifts that they were born to give. Safety and comfort are the gifts that five-sensory individuals who bond as couples were born to give each other and their children. Authentic power is the gift that multisensory humans were born to give to themselves and to Life. Both gifts require commitment and courage, but creating authentic power is more complex than surviving.

A five-sensory female looks for a partner who can protect and provide for her and her children. This is the role of the Old Male. A five-sensory male looks for a partner who can bear and raise his children. This is the role of the Old Female. These five-sensory roles are determined by culture and the requirements of survival. A multisensory female who pursues authentic power can provide for herself. She is competent in her physical and social endeavors, and she chooses her roles in her partnerships. She does not require a partner to protect and provide for her and her children, if she chooses to have children. She is a New Female. A multisensory male who pursues authentic power is emotionally aware, sensitive, and caring for the young, the old, and the ill. He does not require a partner to bring warmth and love into his life. He is warm and loving. This is a New Male.

Old Males and Old Females bond in marriage. New Males and New Females bond in spiritual partnership. Because spiritual partnership is new to the human experience and not yet part of cultural conventions, many New Females and New Males marry to express their love for each other and commitment to growing spiritually together. They participate in the transformation of the archetype of Marriage into the archetype of Spiritual Partnership. Marriage is an ancient bond that was designed for the Old Male and the Old Female. It creates a natural division of labor and mutually beneficial collaborations to support their survival and safety. Relationship between equals for the purpose of spiritual growth was far too advanced a concept to be included in the archetype of Marriage.

New Males and New Females look for partners to share the experiences of spiritual growth and to support one another in creating them. Like a seafarer preparing to embark on a long and challenging journey that beckons, both the New Female and the New Male look for a fellow voyager with commitment to his or her spiritual growth, courage to take responsibility for his or her experiences and heal frightened parts of his or her personality, and compassion for himself or herself and others. They look for the ability to communicate and act consciously instead of unconsciously. In short, they look for a partner to support them in creating authentic power and whom they can support in creating authentic power.

New Males and New Females are emerging everywhere, including in marriages. When an Old Female in a marriage becomes a New Female, the Old Male will transform into a New Male or the marriage will break apart. The inexplicable (and unacceptable to him) changes in his wife will dismay and deeply disturb the Old Male. He will feel that she is breaking her agreement to support his children and care for his home. The Old Female he married agreed to those terms. The New Female is imprisoned by them. If the Old Male stretches himself (challenges the frightened parts of his personality) to a more accurate perception of her changes as healthy instead of dysfunctional, their marriage will transform into a spiritual partnership. If he does not, he will look for another Old Female to provide what he needs.

For example, a wife decided to study architecture when her children were in grade school. Her husband was shaken at first but then began to see new and engaging aspects to the woman he married as she became clear in her intention to study architecture and in her love for him at the same time. His anger turned into curiosity and then into admiration. Her journey into creating authentic power became a mutually supportive journey with a partner into creating authentic power. That is spiritual partnership.

When a New Male emerges into a marriage, the Old Female will transform into a New Female or the marriage will break apart. The Old Female will be shocked by the inexplicable (and unacceptable to her) changes in her spouse. She will feel that he is breaking his agreement to support her and her children and care for her home. If she does not stretch herself (challenge the frightened parts of her personality) to a more accurate perception of his changes as spiritual growth instead of dysfunction, she will look for another Old Male.

An acquaintance with a tenured position at a university, for example, left his teaching career and the security it provided to become a writer. His wife could not understand his decision, and they separated. She felt that he had betrayed his agreement with her, and she wanted their agreement honored. The Old Male made the agreement. The New Male has different potential, more creativity, new goals to pursue, and unexpected gifts to give. Their marriage could have evolved into a spiritual partnership, but the Old Female did not understand or want that and refused to change.

When an Old Female in a marriage becomes a New Female, and an Old Male in a marriage becomes a New Male, their marriage becomes a spiritual partnership and they participate in the transformation of the archetype of Marriage into the new archetype of Spiritual Partnership. In other words, the only marriages that can now support the evolution of humankind are those that are spiritual partnerships.

Spiritual partners stay together because of their choices to grow spiritually (challenge frightened parts of their personalities and cultivate loving parts of their personalities), not because they have a history of being together or have children together. This is very different from five-sensory individuals who remain in a marriage indefinitely because of their fears—of not being able to survive without the other, of not being worthy of love, of not having the strength or courage to begin anew, of being abused, or of leaving the familiarity of their painful power struggles.

Continually refusing to challenge frightened parts of the personality causes a spiritual partnership to dissolve. If one spiritual partner continually refuses to challenge his anger or need to watch pornography, for example, his spiritual growth is not possible, and the reason for the partnership ceases to exist. If the other partner continually refuses to challenge her need to overeat or shop, the same thing happens. They may love one another, but love alone is not enough to keep them together. Spiritual partners bond in order to create authentic power and help one another create authentic power. If one chooses repeatedly to indulge frightened parts of his or her personality instead of challenge them, no vow can keep them together.

Since individuals evolve spiritually at different times and at different rates, most individuals will bond as a couple with more than one spiritual partner in the course of his or her life. This creates a new environment for children. The "nuclear" family that now confines the love and support that children can receive (and expect to receive) to a single home and set of parents will give way to larger extended families that care for many children, provide for the well-being of many children, and love many children. Each "nuclear family" is as difficult to break into as it is to break out of. Five-sensory parents focus on their children to the exclusion of other children, with the result that all children experience their world as safe and caring only in their own home with their own parents, and they carry that sense of danger and of lack of caring away from home with them when they leave it, look for others to create it with, and contribute the same experience in more children.

Children run from strangers, and strangers are reluctant to show affection to unknown children of unknown parents. Assumption of danger is always present because the safety of their children is exceedingly difficult for two parents to insure, but it is less difficult for four parents, less still for eight parents, and virtually guaranteed when all whom their children encounter look upon them as their own children and treasure them as their own children. Eventually humankind will cocreate ways that are appropriate and feasible to care for all children, provide for the well-being of all children, and love all children. Until now, the "Human Family" has remained an empty term, but a cherished one because it promises the potential of relationships of harmony, cooperation, sharing, and reverence for Life that are shared by all, unbound by five-sensory cultural and religious requirements, and treasured by all.

This is not possible when a parent uses a child to satisfy frightened parts of his or her personality. A father, for example, who "takes great pride" in the athletic accomplishments of his child will not "take great pride" in the accomplishments of his neighbor's child, unless frightened parts of his personality also use the accomplishments of his neighbor's child to feel safe and worthy. Will the gold medal that a stranger's child wins fill you with the same satisfaction as the gold medal that your child wins? Will the applause that a neighbor's child receives for a flawless violin recital gratify you as much as the applause that your child receives for a sensational performance? Will it gratify you at all?

Conversely, when frightened parts of the personality of a parent lash out in the pain of powerlessness, targeting children (and spouse), their children grow up in a world in which no safety exists, and they carry these experiences with them when they leave their family, lash out in powerlessness against others (including their own children and spouse), and create those experiences in more children.

The remedy for these painful experiences and the perpetuation of them is authentic power. Social policies and government programs cannot eradicate fear. They can feed fear and cultivate experiences of powerlessness, but they cannot heal them or their sources. Only creating authentic power can do that, and only spiritual partners can support one another and their children, if they have children, in creating authentic power.

For example, a husband and wife had different views on how to manage their finances. He was conservative and wanted to be careful about spending. She was less careful, and this led to conflict. He would question her spending. She would feel disempowered and resented asking him about spending small amounts. They both felt like victims—he of her (to him) thoughtless spending and she of his (to her) obsessive control. As their marriage transformed into a spiritual partnership they began to see each other more as equals and the causes of their fear and anger as frightened parts of their personalities instead of their finances. He saw that if he was angry or frightened about spending, it was a frightened part of his personality. She saw that her fear of being controlled was a frightened part of her personality. They are now able to talk about their finances without all of the painful and hurtful emotional exchanges that previously accompanied their discussions and to challenge frightened parts of their personalities when they become active. Using the Spiritual Partnership Guidelines to create authentic power has changed this aspect of their partnership, and they are changing other aspects of it in the same way.

Five-sensory couples begin their journey together with intense experiences of powerlessness called romantic attraction.

One individual sees in another certain qualities that he admires but (he thinks) lacks. An attraction becomes noticeable and then grows stronger. Even when the attraction appears to be only sexual, it is much more than that. It is attraction to the possibility of permanent release from the pain of powerlessness. Romantic attraction includes sexual attraction and, in addition, a euphoric sense of well-being. Each of the individuals feels more intelligent, sexual, beautiful or handsome, and worthy. The other appears to be the cause of these blissful and exciting experiences. They say to each other, "You complete me," "You make my life worthwhile," or "I have been looking for you for years." Actually, they have been searching for self-value and safety all their lives, and the possibility of finding it through another is exhilarating. It is also delusion.

Savior searching is a means of avoiding the pain of powerlessness. Romantic attraction is the experience of finding a savior. The loneliness, feeling of inadequacy, self-doubt, self-loathing, longing to be lovable and loved, and needing to love as well as be loved momentarily disappear when the "right" individual appears. Finding that individual is not the end of these torments any more than alcohol or drugs, and the relationship of that person to these torments is identical to the relationship of alcohol and drugs to any torment—a temporary anesthetic.

No savior can indefinitely mask the frightened parts of her personality from the one who is saved or from herself. Both individuals in every romantic attraction play the role of the one who is saved. Eventually, anger, emotional withdrawal, jealousy, and more appear in the previously ideal relationship. Money or sex is used to entice the other in moments of fear. Expectations are not met and disappointment follows. Cracks in the illusion widen until both individuals become visible to the other as they are—personalities with frightened parts to be healed and loving parts to be cultivated.

These dynamics appear in heterosexual relationships and same-sex relationships. The choices of love instead of fear, authentic power instead of external power, joy instead of happiness are not gender-based. They are human-based, and the entire human experience is shifting from the fear-oriented pursuit of external power and happiness to the love-oriented creation of authentic power and joy.

Multisensory couples begin their journey by creating authentic power. Individuals who are creating authentic power (using the Spiritual Partnership Guidelines) attract others who are doing the same (Universal Law of Attraction), even if those others have not heard of *spiritual partnership*. Among those they attract and are attracted to, different spiritual partnerships will come into being. Some will be with coworkers, others with neighbors, others with family members, and others with friends. When two individuals recognize each other as potential spiritual partners and choose roles in a partnership that are appropriate to each, a two-person spiritual partnership comes into being. When they choose to live together, or bring children into the Earth school, they form the type of spiritual partnership that is replacing marriage as humankind becomes multisensory.

There is no difference between the purpose and dynamics of this kind of spiritual partnership and the purpose and dynamics of spiritual partnerships among family members, friends, and coworkers. All are partnerships between equals for the purpose of spiritual growth, and in each the partners stay together as long as they grow together, choose their roles, and say what they most fear will destroy their partnership. The roles that they choose for themselves define their partnerships in unique ways and determine the nature of their intimacy and experiences with one another.

To attract potential spiritual partners, create authentic power. There is no other way. The pursuit of external power attracts individuals who are doing the same, and spiritual partnerships are not possible between individuals who are manipulating and controlling one another. Looking for an individual to "complete you," for example, or provide you security, sex, or comfort will attract only individuals who intend to use you in the same way. A spiritual partnership between two multisensory individuals who are committed to creating authentic power together as a couple is entirely different from a marriage between two five-sensory individuals in a lifelong pursuit of external power. The spiritual partnership joins the multisensory individuals as equals for the purpose of spiritual growth for as long as both create authentic power.

Individuals in these partnerships do not see themselves as destined to be together, although many recognize the appropriateness of a relationship that their souls planned prior to incarnation if certain conditions came into being. They do not see each other as the only possible partners in each other's lives, but as the most appropriate for healing the pain of powerlessness that confines each of them and exploring together the depths of their love.

They see every individual as a "soul mate"—a fellow student in the Earth school like themselves, a fellow voyager with whom they have experienced fear and love in many different ways and in many different places and times, and have now come together again. They do not ask themselves, "Is this my soul mate? How will I know?" They remind themselves, "This is my soul mate. How will I relate?"

38

Soul Summary

SPIRITUAL PARTNERSHIPS—WHO

- You can create spiritual partnerships with family members, friends, coworkers, and with another individual as a couple.
- Interactions between parents and children offer the most potential for spiritual growth.
- They are also the most difficult.
- Friends who are interested in spiritual growth naturally become spiritual partners.
- Creating authentic power and spiritual partnerships in a workplace contributes to the transformation of commerce.
- New Males and New Females naturally form spiritual partnerships.
- Spiritual partnerships between New Males and New Females are replacing marriages between Old Males and Old Females.

This is the last of the Soul Summaries. If they have been helpful, experiment with creating your own when you recognize something to be important for your spiritual growth—when an insight expands your perception and understanding or love removes you from fear. Write down your experience and why it is important to you. Keep your Soul Summaries where you can find them, and read them until they are recorded in your heart and you no longer need notes.

I hope that by now Mom (and you, also) are creating authentic power and spiritual partnerships. If not, read this book again starting with the prologue—Change, Possibilities, Power.

Epilogue
More to Come . . .

W hat will happen when *billions* of multisensory individuals each access the wisdom and compassion of the Universe in their own ways, filtering them through their unique individual and collective experiences, and experiment with applying them? How can so many different perceptions and activities serve the evolution of humanity and support Life on the Earth? Religions have taught us the deadly consequences of pitting one understanding of compassion and wisdom against another—both the compassion and wisdom are lost and only competing understandings remain, banners to rally troops in the never-ending battle against those with different understandings, different banners. It matters not whether the image of Christ, Krishna, Buddha, Muhammad, or Moses flies on the banner. In every instance blood—human blood—flows in the name of compassion and wisdom.

What distorts a message of wisdom and compassion so hideously that brothers and sisters kill one another for it? Where there is wisdom there is no fear. Where there is compassion there is love. Wisdom and compassion together illuminate pathways to harmony, cooperation, sharing, and reverence for Life. Who kills for harmony, cooperation, sharing, and reverence for Life? No one who longs for them. Who kills for his or her understanding of wisdom and compassion? That is another story—the religious history of humankind. Only fear can distort a message of wisdom and compassion into a reason—and a need—to destroy other messages and messengers. When the message is one of wisdom and compassion, irony and hypocrisy become indistinguishable.

This irony lies at the heart of every religious movement and raises a red flag of warning for all to see—even compassion and wisdom can be used to justify the pursuit of external power. Five-sensory humans do not recognize the difference between a message and the intention for sharing the message. They assume that if the message is one of compassion and wisdom, sharing it must be a compassionate and wise act. Multisensory humans know otherwise. Five-sensory individuals carry their banners, each proclaiming the unsurpassed benefits of their messages, into battle. They understand power as the ability to manipulate and control, and they intend to acquire it. When they encounter individuals with different banners proclaiming the (sometimes identical) benefits of their message, they lose sight of the benefits and focus on the challenge to their message.

Propagating the message, not creating the benefits, becomes the goal and the means to accomplish it are frequently as lethal as they are ugly. The carnage, brutality, wrenching dislocation, unfathomable suffering, and endless cruelty imposed by one religion upon another in the name of compassion and wisdom (and unsurpassed benefits) fill page after page, chapter after chapter, in the book of five-sensory human history. That book is coming to an end. The final chapters are being written, and we as a collective are writing them.

Multisensory humans look for the intention first and the action second. They know that intention—not action—creates consequences. A message of compassion and wisdom delivered with neither will not bring compassion or wisdom into the Earth school no matter how many times it is delivered. On the contrary, each time the intention to manipulate and control is manifest in the Earth school, more pain results. Preaching prejudice, bigotry, superiority, or violence from a pulpit—however righteously proposed—is the same as presenting cigarettes as a cure for lung cancer. Righteous delivery has no effect. Righteous justification has no effect. Righteously documented evidence has no effect. The cancer grows. The prejudice, bigotry, superiority, and violence spread.

No message can change these things, because they are not created with messages but by intentions. No matter what the message, the intention for sharing it determines the consequences that sharing creates. From the perspective of the five senses, sharing a message requires concepts, images, or music. Intentions are irrelevant. For example, Nazi scientists developed (by sharing concepts) the V2 rocket and advanced fighter and bomber aircraft that could have enabled a new era of transportation linking people and cultures in spectacular ways but that instead enabled the devastating bombardment of London. The Allies devastated Germany with their own ingenious creations that could instead have benefited humanity. Tens of millions of individuals lost their lives. Tens of millions more suffered. Intentions create definite and inevitable consequences. An intention and its consequence can never be separated.

Five-sensory humans say, "By their actions we will know them." Multisensory humans know, "By their intentions we will know them." All of us recognize a tree by its fruit. Only an orange tree can produce oranges. Only an apricot tree can produce apricots. Only the intention to create harmony, cooperation, sharing, and reverence for Life can create harmony, cooperation, sharing, and reverence for Life. Only the intention to pursue external power can create violence and destruction. In other words, from a multisensory perspective, sharing involves much more than concepts, images, and music. What you share and the life you live are identical. "What I do," said Gandhi, "is my religion." We know Gandhi's intentions by his fruits—the nonviolent liberation of an entire subcontinent from brutal colonial occupation, the lived advocacy of the power of love, the demonstrated effectiveness of love, the declaration of love at the moment of his death.

When colleagues complained that Muslims would benefit from Gandhi's intentions, Gandhi (a Hindu) exclaimed, "I am Muslim!" No one doubted that he meant it. His message and intention were identical. The message was love. The intention was love. The result was love on a scale and in a form that surprised the world. In the end, British soldiers on departing troop ships cheered cheering Indians at the dock. How could this have come to be? What message of compassion delivered from a pulpit could have created it? What message of wisdom proclaimed by the devout could have created it?

In this time of overlapping evolutionary modalities—one of them obsolete and counterproductive (the pursuit of external power) and the other emerging and necessary (authentic power)—the verifiable relationship between intention and experience is displacing the illusory relationship between message and experience. No message of love that is not motivated by love can create the experience of love. It can create sentimentality, entitlement, righteousness, and a sense of superiority, but it cannot create the experience of love. Only the intention of love can do that. As we become multisensory, the connection between intention and consequence becomes unmistakable, regardless of the message. How can the intention to love your neighbor, for example, create brutal conflicts between Protestants and Catholics in Northern Ireland? How can hatred of your neighbor not?

The world now pivots on a point and that point is in you. Will you choose to learn wisdom through love and trust or through fear and doubt? When a frightened part of your personality is active, will you challenge it or indulge it? The depths of hopelessness, helplessness, powerlessness are the most painful experiences in the Earth school, and each directs your attention to a frightened part of your personality. Will you have the courage to experience, challenge, and heal it, or will you mask the pain of it with outrage, overeating, judgment of yourself or others, alcohol, sex, drugs, revenge, workaholism, and so forth? Your options appear countless, but there are actually only two—love and fear.

The era of choosing for others, persuading others, convincing others, and converting others has been replaced by a new era in which those same endeavors are profoundly counterproductive. They backfire in big ways. The new era requires distinguishing love from fear in yourself, choosing between them for yourself, and assuming responsibility for the consequences that your choices create. The era of telling others what is best for them and coercing others into what is best for them is over. The era of consulting your intuition and allowing others to consult theirs has arrived. The era of holy righteousness, justifiable outrage, entitlement, and disregard for the processes of others is over. The era of listening to others and creating with the intentions of the soul is here, and it is challenging.

How can you honor the intentions of others when they conflict with your own? How can competing understandings of compassion and wisdom coexist in the human family without tearing it apart? How can they exist in you and your friend without tearing you apart? Five-sensory humans seek to eliminate conflict by manipulating, dominating, or vanquishing others, imposing external power upon them until they conform or perish. "The only good Indian is a dead Indian." "Better dead than red." They do not see one another as brothers and sisters, except those who agree with their understandings, values, and intentions. They see instead savages (as American settlers saw Indians), infidels (as attackers of the World Trade Center saw the people in it and as Christian crusaders saw Muslims), national security threats (for example, enemies in the "war on terror"), vermin (Rwandan Hutus saw Rwandan Tutsis as cockroaches), or rodents (as Nazis saw Jews). The examples are as many as the fears that separate friends, cultures, nations, and religions.

Multisensory humans see fear as the source of conflicts,

not competing understandings and not actions, even abhorrent ones. The futility of fighting fear with fear is visible to them. It increases fear in the world, not diminishes it. It feeds conflict like new wood on a bonfire. Righteousness, rage, revenge, and all other forms of warfare—interpersonal, intercultural, interreligious, and international—are flights from the pain of powerlessness into the pursuit of external power, unconscious creations of hellish realms devoid of compassion and wisdom. Multisensory humans see others as fellow souls that sometimes have frightened parts of their personalities active; students in the Earth school like themselves whose lives are as difficult, complex, and painful as their own; individuals who, like themselves, are learning to create with compassion and wisdom.

An absolute truth is true for all. For example, the Universal Law of Cause and Effect is an absolute truth. If you live by the sword you will die by the sword. If you are loving to others, others will love you. Even if you do not like the language in which an absolute truth is expressed—for example, karma or the Golden Rule—or you do not agree with it, there is a kernel in an absolute truth that everyone can recognize as true. At the very least, an absolute truth can do no harm.

A relative truth is true for you, but it may not be true for others. For example, "the Jews are God's chosen people," "Jesus Christ is our Lord and Savior," "Vishnu is the Destroyer of the World," and many more are relative truths. "Life is nasty, brutish, and short" (Thomas Hobbes), "I think, therefore I am" (René Descartes), and countless other philosophical, theological, emotional, and psychological truths are relative—accurate and definitive for some individuals, and inaccurate, fantastical, or heretical for others. Relative truths define piety and blasphemy something like customs define good and bad manners, but there is a big difference between a relative truth and good manners. Violating good manners is not lethal, but millions of humans have been killed for disagreeing with a relative truth of others.

Individuals impose relative truths on one another with judgment, anger, withdrawal, jealousy, etc., as well as brute force. Religions, nations, and cultures impose them with sanctions, policies, dogmas, and brutality, such as the Spanish Inquisition (death by torture) of non-Catholics and the ruthless, methodical massacre of six million Jews (and millions of other non-Aryans) in Nazi Germany. Proclaiming a relative truth to be absolute is the pursuit of external power. Every religion does it. Every homicide and genocide results from it. All violence comes from it. Only you can stop it, and only in yourself. Only you can challenge and heal the frightened parts of your personality that pursue external power, and only you can cultivate the loving parts. Only you can create in yourself the world that you long to see.

The Spiritual Partnership Guidelines show you how. They lead you, step-by-step, from unempowerment to empowerment, from a life of fear and pain to a life of love and joy. The Spiritual Partnership Guidelines prevent you from imposing your fear on others and help you recognize when others are imposing theirs. They help you shift your perceptions from frightened to loving and to create consciously and constructively. Following the Spiritual Partnership Guidelines insures that you will honor the understandings of others whether or not you agree with them and prevents your disagreements, when they occur, from becoming contaminated with fear.

The Spiritual Partnership Guidelines move you beyond the influence of cultures, customs, and religions. They free you from the restraints of your fears (frightened parts of your personality) and the fears (frightened parts of the personality) of others and show you how to move through your life with an empowered heart without attachment to the outcome. The Spiritual Partnership Guidelines enable you to do your best in every circumstance.

As you free yourself from the frightened parts of your personality, you become able to create harmony, cooperation, sharing, and reverence for Life because you choose to, because you decide to contribute to Life instead of exploit life regardless of what others choose, because you want the humbleness, forgiveness, clarity, and Love of authentic power more than you want the painful, endless roller coaster of fear and want, want and fear, because the gifts that you give to yourself are the gifts that you give to others at the same time.

This is the moment of transformation, of spiritual growth exploding through your life, destroying your old goals and old ways of achieving them and replacing them with the exhilarating, healing, fulfilling potential of authentic power. The more you create authentic power, the more you create the potential for spiritual partnership. There is no limit to the number of spiritual partnerships that you can cocreate, because there is no limit to the number of potential spiritual partners. My dream is an eight-billion-person partnership between equals for the purpose of spiritual growth. What is your dream?

The impact of spiritual partnership is far-reaching and the potential of it is vast. If you want substantive, deep, and significant relationships in your life, you are already feeling that potential. If you are excited about living your life with compassion and wisdom instead of defending your understanding of compassion and wisdom, you are already feeling that potential. If your heart is opening to yourself and others, or you think it might be, you are feeling that potential.

A new light is appearing in the night sky.

Sunrise is coming.

An Invitation to Join Gary Zukav and Linda Francis at the Seat of the Soul Institute

My spiritual partner Linda Francis and I founded the Seat of the Soul Institute in 1999 to share, teach, learn, and celebrate with dedicated persons who seek continuing growth throughout life.

Simply stated, our vision is to create a world in which spiritual development becomes the highest priority—with lives enriched by alignment of the personality and the soul . . . with individuals courageously pursuing and discovering unexplored realms of human potential . . . with couples and collectives bonded through love and common commitment to spiritual growth.

At the Institute we also focus on expanding interpersonal awareness and how to achieve healthier, more collaborative and enriching relationships. We've designed some unique programs and events to support you and those you cherish in creating *authentic power* and transformational *spiritual partnerships*.

I invite you to venture forward by joining our web community. You'll discover how we expand the teachings and insights in this book in ways that aware and loving interactions can achieve. You'll meet some inspiring, incredible people who share your goals and dreams. You'll find out how our many activities and programs can support you even more as you seek renewal, growth, creativity, and infinitely loving relationships.

We hope you'll consider becoming part of our ever-expanding spiritual partnership community of individuals making personal development and cocreative spiritual relationships their highest priorities.

You can join our community by visiting www.seatofthesoul .com. Linda and I look forward to cocreating the next chapters of our journeys . . . with you . . . and soon.

Love,

Gary Zukav

Welcome.
Please join us at
www.seatofthesoul.com.

Acknowledgments

I am very grateful to Linda Francis, whose constant love and inspiration nurture me and whose many contributions to this book have made it ever so much more practical and useful. I am grateful to my spiritual partners everywhere, and especially to the participants in the Authentic Power Program of the Seat of the Soul Institute, whose commitment, courage, compassion, and conscious communications and actions so often inspire me. I am also grateful to my editor, Gideon Weil, whose suggestions have made this book more personal and inviting.

Index